"Fazlur Rahman is a wonderful storyteller. I was immediately drawn in by the vivid characters, touched by their plights and by the author's depth of compassion."

—Jonathan Balcombe, bestselling author of
What a Fish Knows and *Super Fly*

"Cancer touches countless lives worldwide. As a cancer researcher, I applaud Dr. Rahman's effort to make cancer biology accessible to everyone in *Our Connected Lives*. As a physician, I appreciate how his thoughtful stories illuminate the practice of cancer medicine—not just by revealing the struggles patients and doctors face, but also by highlighting the importance of treating patients as people rather than cases. The lessons in this book are instructive for us all: cancer patients and their loved ones, general readers as well as the members of the medical profession."

—Hagop M. Kantarjian, MD, Professor and Chair, Department of Leukemia; Samsung Distinguished University Chair in Cancer Medicine; MD Anderson Cancer Center, University of Texas

"Dr. Fazlur Rahman's *Our Connected Lives: Caring for Cancer Patients in Rural Texas* is a must-read, flush with all the richness of human life in the face of illness. In these pages, the cancer doctor walks alongside his patients through the difficult conversations, complex medical decisions, losses and triumphs that cancer brings. Dr. Rahman's intense empathy for his West Texas patients vivifies these pages, and drives him to provide excellent, diligent, humane care. Any reader who wants to know what cancer is like from the other side—the doctor's side—will be enlightened to find in Dr. Rahman's stories a testimony to how deeply doctors care for our patients and indeed how connected we all are, in the end. If you have doubted whether doctors actually care not only for patients but about them as human beings, this book will change you. It shows how the best doctors among us are, and how we all ought to be."

—Rachel Pearson, MD, PhD, Humanities Director, Charles E. Cheever, Jr. Center for Medical Humanities and Ethics; Joe R. and Teresa Lozano Long Distinguished Professor in Bioethics; author, *No Apparent Distress: A Doctor's Coming of Age on the Front Lines of American Medicine*

"The renowned clinician Dr. William Osler, considered the 'Father of Internal Medicine,' observed: 'The good physician treats the disease; the great physician treats the patient who has the disease.'

Fazlur Rahman is not only a great physician; this remarkable man is also a wonderful writer.

From his humble beginnings in what is now Bangladesh (and for this story I highly recommend his cultural memoir, *The Temple Road*), and throughout his post-graduate training in internal medicine and oncology in New York and Houston, it took amazing fortitude and faith for Dr. Rahman to find his way to San Angelo, Texas. There he garnered the love and respect of its citizens through his delivery of high-quality primary and specialty care over many decades.

How he accomplished this is the main thrust of this memoir. Every turn this writer takes—into medical science, the evolution of oncological treatments, the intricacies of doctor-patient-family relationships—serves to enlighten and enhance this story. This physician's dedicated attentiveness to the daily, then yearly, then career-long practice of patient-centered 'connected' medicine is rare in America's fractured health system today, and we are all the poorer for it.

With this book, Dr. Rahman joins the ranks of other great physician writers: Anton Chekhov, William Carlos Williams, Richard Selzer, Oliver Sacks, and Abraham Verghese, among others. You will not be able to put this book down. And when the last page is turned, you may wonder where you might find someone like this author to care for you. I know I did."

—Jerald Winakur, MD, MACP, FRCP
Author of *Memory Lessons: A Doctor's Story* and *Human Voices Wake Us*

"The story of each of these five unforgettable women and men makes a powerful reading. These are mesmerizing and page-turner tales, making us genuinely concerned about the lives of those individuals with cancer. But their stories are also relevant to other people whether they have cancer or not."

—Kanti Rai, MD, Winner of the ASH Wallace H. Coulter Award for Lifetime Achievement in Hematology

OUR
CONNECTED
LIVES

OUR CONNECTED LIVES

CARING FOR CANCER PATIENTS IN RURAL TEXAS

FAZLUR RAHMAN

TEXAS TECH UNIVERSITY PRESS

This book is typeset in EB Garamond. The paper used in this book meets the minimum requirements of ANSI/NISO Z39.48-1992 (R1997). ♾

Designed by Hannah Gaskamp
Cover design by Hannah Gaskamp

Library of Congress Cataloging-in-Publication Data

Names: Rahman, Fazlur (Oncologist), author. Title: Our Connected Lives: Caring for Cancer Patients in Rural Texas / Fazlur Rahman. Description: Lubbock, Texas: Texas Tech University Press, [2024] | Includes bibliographical references and index. | Summary: "One of the first full-time oncologists in West Texas reflects on a life of service to his patients"—Provided by publisher.
Identifiers: LCCN 2024022248 (print) | LCCN 2024022249 (ebook) |
ISBN 978-1-68283-222-6 (cloth; alk. paper) | ISBN 978-1-68283-223-3 (paperback; alk. paper)
ISBN 978-1-68283-224-0 (ebook)
Subjects: MESH: Physician-Patient Relations | Neoplasms—therapy | Patient Care—methods | Oncologists—psychology | Texas | Personal Narrative Classification: LCC RC277.T4 R34 2024 (print) | LCC RC277.T4 (ebook) | NLM QZ 200 | DDC 616.99/4009764—dc23/eng/20240726
LC record available at https://lccn.loc.gov/2024022248
LC ebook record available at https://lccn.loc.gov/2024022249

Texas Tech University Press
Box 41037
Lubbock, Texas 79409-1037 USA
800.832.4042
ttup@ttu.edu

To:

—Jahanara (Ara): for all her love and sustenance
—Bazlur Rahman: for being an inspiration in creative work
—Amina, Adam, Abran, Amira, Amala, and Zayan: for pointing us toward a better world

"Through chances various, through all
vicissitudes, we make our way . . ."
—VIRGIL, *THE AENEID*

". . . and I think of each life as a flower, as common
as a field daisy, and as singular . . ."
—MARY OLIVER, "WHEN DEATH COMES"

CONTENTS

CONTENTS

OUR
CONNECTED
LIVES

INTRODUCTION

T o be a cancer doctor and to write the stories of my patients once seemed improbable. So how did I become an oncologist in the first place? It began with my mother, and later, with a nine-year-old boy named Tobi who had osteogenic sarcoma, a deadly bone tumor.

I grew up in the 1950s in a small village in what is now Bangladesh. At age seven, a malicious parasitic illness called kala-azar almost extinguished my life. This happened at the worst time of my existence, when I was coping with unbearable grief: just months before my illness, my mother had suddenly died from unrelenting hemorrhage during childbirth. Right before her labor pain started, she had asked me to give her a glass of water to drink, and she quenched her thirst in front of me. A few hours later, she was gone. Bewilderment and sorrow overwhelmed me. I had been a sensitive and sickly child since birth, and my mother was my protective shield.

Mother had seen a lot of suffering and death in her short years on this earth, including the loss of her first child and other children in the village, and of family members and friends. They had succumbed to cholera and other epidemics that plagued the population of the Indian subcontinent at the time. Most died without any medical care. When I was about six, malaria took away Mother's younger brother, a village schoolteacher. She loved him with all her heart, and his death crushed her. "He was so young and so good. Why did he have to leave that early?" Mother would moan time and again. She would often gaze into my eyes and confide wistfully, "Someday you will be a doctor, Fazlur, and help people." Her words were etched in my mind from that tender age.

I was a scion of a respected mullah family whose old money had vanished but whose name still mattered. My paternal grandmother, a strong-willed widow, wanted to send me to a madrasa, an Islamic school, to enhance the clan's name. Among other things, people looked to us for spiritual guidance. She was the family matriarch and held sway in that male-dominated culture. But the madrasa education didn't have a strong curriculum in science and mathematics, and this shortfall would have forever closed the door to medical school.

My luck, however, prevailed this time. My grandmother treated my mother as her own daughter, and to honor my mother's memory, she abandoned her own desire and let my father enroll me in Benapole School to begin my standard education. I excelled throughout my school years and qualified for college. Though I was a science student aiming for medicine, I loved poetry and literature in English and Bengali, my mother tongue, and spent more of my time reading those subjects. This had an unintended effect: I scored better in the liberal arts subjects than in science. This lopsided result wasn't taken very favorably by the admissions committee at Dhaka Medical College, the best medical school, where I applied, and for which there was intense competition for admission. Some committee members felt that I was only half-heartedly interested in medicine and that my actual interest lay in poetry and literature. Fortunately, others on the committee saw something in me and found that my science scores were still competitive enough to give me a chance.

Yet, that didn't end the challenges in my education. Our courses in medical school began with the dissection of a cadaver. But defiling the dead was a sacrilege to my grandmother. As I put my knife on the cadaver—an elderly man—my hand shook, and I prayed to God to forgive me. I was only seventeen and racked with inner conflict: was I in the right calling? I had no one to turn to, for there was no counseling in medical school. I coped on my own by thinking of my dear mother; abandoning her wish was inconceivable. In this way, I calmed my turmoil and completed the course.

After two years of basic sciences, it was time to learn bedside medicine for three years. My earlier struggles with medicine resurfaced. When I saw the poor and destitute patients at Dhaka Medical College Hospital, the only charity hospital in that vast megalopolis, I was distressed by their anguish—and worse, by their untimely deaths. "What difference am I making in this sea of suffering?" I wondered. But it was my luck that I came under the influence of a brilliant teacher and clinician, Professor S. M. Rab. He noticed my struggles, and one day he called me to his office. "Look at the brighter side of medicine," he said. "We cure many common infections like typhoid and amebiasis, and we lessen the medical misery of others. Don't forget Fleming's discovery of penicillin and what it has done to eliminate near-fatal strep throat in children, and the rest. Medicine will always improve for the better, and you want to be a part of that." Before penicillin, strep throat infection, among other complications, induced rheumatic fever, which was the single greatest cause of disabling damage to heart valves, leading to heart failure.

The penicillin story also hit close to home. As a sickly child, I had taken my share of this revolutionary antibiotic. Alexander Fleming was widely known and was our medical god. He died in 1955, only seven years before I entered medical school. Professor Rab's examples and doings inspired me and pulled me through. And I continued my medical journey with renewed interest.

Later, Tobi, the boy with sarcoma of the thigh bone, came into my life in the surgical ward. His cancer progressed while he waited for an operation to amputate his cancerous thigh, a procedure that rarely controlled the tumor. But at that time and place, it was the sole treatment option. At first, his father begged us not to cut off the limb. The boy would be a pitiful invalid, he said. How would he make a living? Which parents would marry their daughter to him? But seeing that his son was getting worse, he finally agreed to the amputation.

Tobi survived the surgery. But a week later, he was struggling for breath. We thought it was due to pulmonary embolism or pneumonia, the usual postoperative complications. It was neither. Tobi had developed rapidly advancing bilateral lung metastasis—the cancer had spread to both lungs and was now devouring them. His father desperately watched his son go downhill. The next day, Tobi clasped his father's hands and took his last gasp. His death was utterly devastating to this poor man, who had to grieve alone. His wife and family lived in a distant village, and they couldn't afford to send Tobi's mother with him.

Tobi's excruciating end stayed with me, as did his agony from intractable bone pain. How helpless I felt when I was unable to give him morphine, the best analgesic, to ameliorate his anguish. Morphine, being a narcotic, had a bad connotation, and it aroused undue fear among the doctors, so they prescribed it reluctantly and in inadequate doses at irregular intervals, and patients were often forced to endure horrendous pain. As a medical student,

I was powerless to change anything. But Tobi compelled me to learn more about cancer and find ways to ease the suffering of its victims. To do that, I needed a postgraduate education.

However, there was an almost insurmountable hurdle in front of me. By now, the country was run by military dictators. A budding doctor mattered little in that regime. I had a superb academic record, graduating in the top ten among the four hundred students across four medical schools. But that didn't count for admission to the new postgraduate institute in Dhaka, which accepted doctors by seniority or based on political connections, regardless of merit. Moreover, there was a five-year waiting list for admission, and even if I waited that long, my chances of acceptance were bleak. I would be languishing without a future. My only option was to leave the country for advanced studies in the UK or the United States.

I researched opportunities in both countries and found that, compared to the British higher education system, the American system was more open to me. All I had to do was to take a US qualifying examination—the Educational Commission for Foreign Medical Graduates (ECFMG) certification—and apply for an internship. I passed the ECFMG and secured an internship at St. John's Hospital in Yonkers, New York, in 1969. That was to be the beginning of my American odyssey. St. John's offered me more than I expected—a stipend, free food and lodging, and my airfare from Dhaka to New York. Subsequently, I did my residency at Long Island Jewish Medical Center and Queens Hospital Center in New York City, then my senior residency and fellowship at Baylor College of Medicine in Houston.

Unlike my student days in Dhaka, where cancer was uncommon, in the US it was the second most common cause of death, just behind cardiovascular disease. In this new setting, my old curiosity about cancer biology was reinforced, and I veered towards the oncology field. Then I read a seminal report, published in 1970, by Dr. Vincent DeVita and his group at the National Cancer Institute. They had potentially cured or had put into remission advanced Hodgkin's lymphoma—a disease that would have killed these patients within a short time—using a four-drug combination chemotherapy termed MOPP.

The "cure" of such advanced cancer was amazing to me. What also drew my interest was how two of the MOPP drugs—Mustargen (nitrogen mustard) and Oncovin—came into use. Nitrogen mustard is derived from poisonous mustard gas. Its original purpose was aimed at killing people, not saving them, for it was developed as a chemical warfare agent, and its anticancer property was accidentally discovered. During World War II, some of the gas was secretly stored in a US cargo ship and harbored in Bari, Italy, for its possible use as a chemical weapon. German bombs exploded the ship, and hundreds of Allied soldiers and civilians were killed or maimed from exposure to the gas. Unfortunately, since neither the crew nor the soldiers knew of this clandestine warfare project, they had no knowledge of its treatment. Autopsies of the victims found damage to their organs and blood cells. Based on this, further research was done, which eventually led to nitrogen mustard, the first chemotherapy drug. Oncovin (vincristine), on the other hand, is an alkaloid extracted from periwinkle plants.

After I finished my fellowship in hematology/oncology, I wanted to make a career in academics and research. But life's practicalities intervened. A week before leaving Bangladesh, I had married a village girl I loved, amid dire circumstances, spurning an arranged bride from an influential urban family. The separation was painful for us. During my training in New York, I worked hard and lived hand-to-mouth and saved money. Eighteen months later, I had accumulated enough funds to bring Jahanara (Ara), my wife, to me, and we had a child. We had both grown up in hardship and scarcity, and I didn't want my Ara to go through that again. But we were short of cash and had no one to ask for financial help, and at the time, the starting academic salary was low. More disconcerting, five of my professors at Baylor whom I admired left academics for private practice. They and a mentor of mine advised me to do the same because of my financial needs. I took their advice, and in July 1975 went to a place where I was needed the most: San Angelo, a city of 70,000 people in far West Texas, 400 miles northwest of Houston. I settled there with my family and practiced cancer medicine for thirty-five years. In retrospect, the move turned out to be auspicious beyond self-sufficiency, for it gave me a chance for deep interactions with my own patients.

I have always been interested in the lives of my patients beyond medicine. But my training years were so hectic that I barely had time to get to know them. Like any doctor in training in those days, I had to regularly rotate to various wards and services in the hospitals. In the process, the patients became almost a blur. However, in private practice in a remote rural town, things were different. I had to take care of all kinds of patients—from farmers, ranchers, and teachers to active and retired soldiers to oil field workers. For years, I was the only oncologist within about a 200-mile radius, and my patients often depended on me for other care outside oncology. Through a combination of diligence and good fortune, I had earned American board certification in three disciplines: Internal Medicine, Hematology, and Oncology. Therefore, I was comfortable doing primary care for my hematologic and oncologic patients if I needed to. This gave me ample opportunity to become familiar with their daily lives and their families. I shared their joys and sorrows. The setting was quite different from the larger academic and cancer centers, where patients are routinely switched from specialty to specialty, even for minor ailments. Moreover, I had been trained at a time when bedside medicine was more valued, and medical technology, though essential for diagnosis and treatment, didn't supersede bedside judgment.

It's not a cliché to say that medicine is a lifelong learning process, and even after more than half a century of being a doctor, my professional life remains full of discovery. And what about those struck by cancer? In my close involvement with them, their multitude of problems besides their cancer came into sharp relief for me. Life doesn't take a break while you are at the clinic. My patients not only had to fight cancer but also cope with everyday living: family and other relationships, career, insurance, bureaucracy, money, and the rest. Surgery, chemotherapy, and radiation didn't solve any of that.

As the years passed, I wrote articles and stories for many influential national and international publications, inserting snippets of the lives of my patients and of my own life with them. In the pages ahead, I narrate the detailed stories of five of them. I chose them because they illuminate the humanity in all of us; reveal courage and resilience in the face of tragedy and setbacks; and show the inner workings of chemotherapy as well as the cancer field. Equally important, the stories tell about how these patients dealt with me as their oncologist, how I learned from them, and how I fought my doubts and difficulties about their treatments.

Moreover, these patients are instructive examples of certain unique aspects of cancer care: surviving against all odds; walking a long path with cancer and still making a daily life; facing the crushing burden of the exorbitant cost of cancer drugs and being forced to decide between saving your own life and having enough for your family to live on; experiencing the vagaries of old age and coping with malignancy; and patients' desire for dignity—dignity that we all want, rich or poor. They speak for cancer patients everywhere, for they all suffer in the same or similar ways, only some more and some less depending on their disease and their means and support.

All of my oncology classmates chose to settle in large cities such as Houston, Dallas, and Phoenix. Medical Oncology, our specialty, was new, so it was in demand then as it is now. At the time, not many doctors wanted to go into cancer care, saying, "It's too depressing." They would rather take cardiology, gastroenterology, and the like.

When I told my colleagues I was going to San Angelo, they first asked me where the place was. Hearing that it was in West Texas, a few said, "Why do you want to go to the boondocks? There's nothing there except oil fields and roughnecks."

How wrong they were. As I look back, I am glad that I chose San Angelo. The kind of intimacy that I developed with my patients and their loved ones would have been difficult in big cities. My family and I became part of the community, and its people became a part of me. Their welfare mattered to me beyond medicine. I believe that all this, in addition to my own suffering in my growing-up years, made me a better doctor.

When my patients achieved remission, I was as gratified as they were. But many didn't, and yet, in the midst of their suffering, they still thanked me for being there for them. The feeling that I was making a difference—however little—in this distant corner of the country gave me more impetus to reaffirm my commitment to care for the sick, and to understand an essential need in medical practice: empathy.

I learned one more life lesson from my professional career in West Texas, and I mention this out of gratitude, not out of hubris. Upon my retirement in 2011, the *San Angelo Standard-Times* ran a front-page story about me, headlined, "Doctor Retires with Love and Respect." If I was awarded love and respect, what more reward could I ask for? It was the simplicity and generosity of the rural, small-town people that bestowed me with these sentiments, despite my failings. Sure, I had to deal with my share of individuals who didn't care for black- or brown-skinned persons, doctor or not, but they were overshadowed by the vast number of good-hearted souls.

PART 1

CLARA: DEFYING THE DOCTORS

CHAPTER 1

Sunrise and sunset are glorious in West Texas. The vastness of its sky makes up for its scarcity of trees and shrubbery. The brilliant glows of its heavens signify hope for a new day in the morning and a new night in the evening. I need hope, day and night, for my patients and me. I am a cancer doctor.

It was another early Monday morning in the hospital, and I was sitting in a quiet corner of the doctors' dining room, drinking tea. But my mind was elsewhere. The night before, my patient, Sandy Oliver, had been admitted again through the ER. She had intractable nausea and vomiting from chemotherapy. I had spent two hours with her in the oncology ward. Once she was stabilized with IV fluid and electrolytes, I went home. She had been fighting breast cancer for four years, and her lung metastasis seemed under control with treatment. But now her cancer had outwitted her and me and spread to her bones and liver. What could I tell her today that I hadn't told her already?

She was only thirty-two years old when the cancer was diagnosed, and she had three small children. Breaking the news was hard. She collapsed on her pillow and sobbed, and her husband looked stunned at her bedside. I couldn't stop my eyes from watering. Sandy and her husband were an inseparable couple. They had fallen in love in high school and later married, and they had stayed as close as they'd been in their student days.

A few weeks after the diagnosis, Sandy was reconciled to her new state. As time went on, her courage and grace astonished and inspired me. "It's not your fault, Doctor," she said to me more than once. In the end, she would leave the world but not my mind.

An internist colleague paged me and broke my trance. "I have an interesting case for you," he said. "She has metastatic cancer, but I don't know where it's coming from. Maybe from the breast."

Whenever I heard the words "an interesting case," my antennae went up. What's interesting for a doctor is bad news for a patient.

The referral from the internist was a thirty-nine-year-old woman named Clara Anderson. She had felt poorly for four months. Her appetite had decreased, so she cut down on her meals and fluids. She lost weight and became dehydrated. She had been admitted to the hospital with severe back pain two days before and was on low-dose morphine.

As I introduced myself at her bedside, she gazed up with sad eyes. "I'm sorry, Doctor," she said. "I look terrible. I can't take care of myself here."

Her remark seemed out of place, given her condition. I thought the morphine had maybe dulled her thinking. Her husband Mark, sitting on the other side of the bed, spoke up.

"I've been begging her to see her doctor. I knew something wasn't right. Then her pain suddenly got worse. That's when she agreed to come to the ER."

The x-rays ordered by her internist showed lesions on the spine and ribs that suggested cancer. As my colleague suspected, at Clara's age, given these findings, breast cancer with bone metastasis—meaning the cancer had spread to the bone—was the most likely diagnosis. I sensed that she didn't know that yet. I hoped she wouldn't be another Sandy Oliver.

Mrs. Anderson was a tall, beautiful woman with well-combed hair, blond and lush, that fell below her shoulders. Her arched eyebrows were penciled in, and her polished nails glistened. The faded, crumpled hospital gown looked incongruous on her. I was amazed how she had managed to be so tidy amid all her troubles. She looked exhausted, but alert, not dulled by the morphine as I had thought.

After getting her history, I did a thorough examination. When I pressed on her lower spine, she winced, "That hurts!" Most important, on palpation, her breasts were normal. But breast cancer still had to be ruled out. To be detectable by examining fingers, a tumor needs to be at least 0.4 inches in size and be located closer to the surface. Her breasts were of moderate size, and the cancer could easily have hidden in their depths.

She remembered that two years earlier, she had felt something on her right breast, and her gynecologist ordered a mammogram. It didn't show any abnormalities. She had ignored the advice to have a follow-up mammogram. I asked her why.

"They flattened my breasts under that damned machine," she said, "and it hurt a lot. The technician said she had to apply that much pressure to get good pictures. My breast got bruised and painful. Once was enough."

Her complaint about the mammogram wasn't unusual, but I couldn't ignore her current findings.

"We're worried you may have a breast tumor," I said. "We need another mammogram."

"They said the same thing when they asked me to have the first one, and they were wrong."

"Things are different now. You weren't sick then and you didn't have bone pain. I'll give you extra pain medicine and talk to our x-ray tech first."

She reluctantly consented, and a day later we had the mammogram. Surprisingly, it showed no suspicious lesions. I ordered a bone scan, which helps to gauge the extent of the bone metastases. This, too, defied my expectations—it was unremarkable.

In clinical practice, if you have a confusing situation, you think like a detective. Abnormal bone x-rays with a normal bone scan pointed to something more sinister—not a breast tumor, but a blood cancer known as multiple myeloma (in short, myeloma or MM). X-rays of Clara's skull showed characteristic damage to the bones called lytic changes, areas eaten up by cancer. But in her case, they were so-called punched-out lesions, like Swiss cheese with incomplete holes—a telltale sign of myeloma. However, breast cancer itself can sometimes cause these kinds of changes, and at the age of thirty-nine, it's ten times more prevalent than myeloma.

Clara's lab tests revealed anemia, high calcium, and poor kidney function. But these findings were of little help because metastatic breast cancer with dehydration can also induce these anomalies. What then—breast cancer or myeloma?

To understand myeloma, one needs to understand a group of proteins in our circulatory system called immunoglobulins or antibodies, which fight infection. They are manufactured by plasma cells, a type of cell in the bone marrow. Unfortunately, cells that keep us alive can also kill us when they turn malignant.

When a plasma cell mutates to become cancerous, it multiplies endlessly like any other cancer, creating its own clones. The clones, in turn, secrete a specific type of abnormal protein termed M protein or monoclonal protein (mono means single).

While normal immunoglobulin proteins help kill bacteria, viruses, and fungi, an M protein has no such ability. To make matters worse, the cancerous protein suppresses the normal ones. Thus, myeloma patients are vulnerable to infections. Moreover, one type of M protein has another destructive habit: it accumulates in the kidneys, damaging them and blocking their function.

Besides producing plasma cells, bone marrow also generates other blood cells that are essential for our survival: white cells (of which plasma cells are a variety), red cells, and platelets. Each group has its own particular function. White cells fight infections along with the immunoglobulins, red cells contain hemoglobin that carries oxygen throughout the body, and platelets facilitate blood clotting. Myeloma, being malignant, overwhelms the production of the normal white cells, red cells, and platelets in the bone marrow.

Clara's high blood calcium could have been a red flag. Cancerous bones can release extra calcium into the circulation, raising its blood level, and this is more common with myeloma than with breast cancer. Common or uncommon, in the end, my hunch was that the root of her ills was myeloma.

But one can't simply act on a hunch with a potentially lethal disease. I needed a solid diagnosis, and to reach that, I had to study the source of her malady. The source, in this case, was the bone marrow (BM) where the malignant plasma cells had originated. Getting a BM sample required a combined procedure known as bone marrow aspiration and biopsy. This is done by inserting a wide-bore needle into a hip bone, then drawing out the marrow with a syringe. After that, a small sample of the marrow core is taken.

Knowing that Clara—she had asked me to call her by her first name—resisted needles, I approached her cautiously about the procedure. In hindsight, I wish I had chosen my words differently, until I had developed more rapport or until I had established the diagnosis.

"Well, Clara, myeloma is a possibility. It's a kind of cancer that starts in the bone marrow, like leukemia."

"Oh God!" she cried out before I could explain further. "Not leukemia. My older sister died of acute leukemia. I was about twelve then."

She hadn't told me about her sister when I first took her history. I believe the omission was more of a defense from a painful memory than from deception. I assured her that she didn't have leukemia, but it did little to mollify her.

"They did too many bone marrows on Laura," she said. "What good did it do? All she got was pain. The treatment almost killed her. I don't want to go through what my sister did. I might as well die and get it over with. I don't want to suffer."

Words have consequences, especially in my work as a cancer doctor. Acute leukemia in adults is a deadly malignancy, and its treatment is harrowing. Clara had ample reason to react the way she did. I had to repair the damage my word "leukemia" had caused.

"Myeloma is much more treatable than acute leukemia," I said, "and it's also easier to treat. All you have to do is to take a few tablets every few weeks, not the strong IV chemotherapy your sister had."

"Then why don't you give me the tablets and see if they'll work?"

"It's still a chemotherapy drug. I can't give it without a firm diagnosis. We have to do the bone marrow for that."

The bone marrow procedure is commonly performed for the evaluation of hematologic (blood-related) diseases. It's done at the bedside, and despite its frequency, it sparks fear in people's minds—more so with Clara because of her sister's ordeal.

The iliac bones—a pair of flat bones on each side of the hip—are one of the biggest reservoirs of the marrow in adults. Each iliac bone has a crest, which is the preferred site for marrow extraction. If you lie on your stomach, you can feel the crest on either side of your lower back.

Clara had more pain in the right crest. That's where I decided to insert my bone marrow needle, the Jamshidi type, named after its inventor, Khosrow Jamshidi.

"Why do you want to push a needle in a place that hurts me already?" she asked. "Can't you do this on the left side?"

She had my sympathy. I explained a paradox in medical evaluation. Because the pathology often lies where the pain is, doctors hurt where they shouldn't be hurting in the first place. In her case, we were more likely to find the abnormal cells on the painful site.

To dull her discomfort, I premedicated her with injections of an analgesic and a local anesthetic. After these took effect, I aspirated about five ccs of marrow and passed it to the lab technician standing next to me. She immediately made slides with the material while I did the bone marrow biopsy. All this together took me only six or seven minutes; by now I had done the procedure more than a hundred times.

For me to access Clara's iliac crest, she had to lie on her stomach. Hence, though she was awake, she couldn't see me. But to reassure her, I described step by step what I was doing. There was one thing, however, that couldn't be helped. Despite the analgesics, the aspiration elicits a brief but sharp pain on the needle site. Clara's pain was worse because it was in a part of the bone that was hurting already.

"You told me you'd try not to hurt me," she complained, "but you did. I had to grit my teeth."

"I didn't mean to. I took all the precautions I could, but your situation is special."

"You call this special?"

"I'm sorry, Clara. I wish there were another way of doing this."

Back in my office lab, I examined the marrow slides under a microscope. As I scanned them, my hope that my hunch could be wrong faded. Her bone marrow had gone haywire, but in a strange way. There were those elegant cells with their bluish hue; how lovely they appeared, dotting the marrow field, like stars studding the night sky. But their elegance and beauty were utterly deceptive, for they were plasma cells with a murderous character. They had taken over most of the marrow and replaced the normal cells. Clara's plasma cell count was 60 percent, or thirty times normal.

A high plasma cell count (plasmacytosis) can also be caused by some nonmalignant conditions, such as cirrhosis of the liver. In these diseases, however, the counts are far lower. Besides, plasmacytosis alone isn't sufficient to meet the criteria for the diagnosis of multiple myeloma. We must also confirm the presence of the monoclonal protein, the M protein, made by these malignant cells.

In 85 percent of myeloma patients, the M protein is present in the blood, but in the remaining 15 percent, it's detected in the urine. Sure enough, Clara's urine sample was awash with the M protein that damages the kidneys. This explained her kidney dysfunction. But this protein wasn't the only thing the malignant cells were responsible for; they were also chewing up her bones, making them lytic and brittle.

I was reluctant to put these things together, knowing what it would mean to Clara's life. She had married early and had children, first a girl and then a boy. "They changed my whole world," she had said to me. "I quit teaching to raise them. Mark is out a lot as an oil field technician. The children have become old enough, and I want to go back to my job. I love teaching, and we could use the money for our kids." She had a rhythm in her days and hope for her family, and she was happy.

Now, with my diagnosis, her life's rhythm and her hoped-for future would not only be disrupted but could be extinguished altogether. Yet, my reluctance couldn't alter the cold facts—myeloma had been confirmed beyond doubt. In addition, with her high M protein and calcium plus her anemia, lytic bones, and poor kidneys, she had the most advanced stage of the disease, stage three. Clara's chances of survival were dismal. She had entered the realm of a pitiless adversary and its treacherous bones.

Brittle bones exact a price. Patients are at constant risk of fractures, at times spontaneous and without warning, and at other times after only minor activity, like getting up from a chair. In the past, hip fractures, in particular, were a menace to these patients. In many cases, it was hard to know what happened first—a fall and then a fracture or the other way around. The fractures were a common cause of disability and death because they were hard to fix. After an operation, the bones wouldn't hold together, or they would simply disintegrate. In the 1970s and 1980s, I had more than one patient suffer this fate. On top of that, relentless pain compounded their misery. Being bedridden worsened their state by making the skeleton still more fragile. Luckily, a new medication, pamidronate, was introduced in about 1999 to heal myeloma bones, the cause of much of the suffering.

I was the bearer of bad news to Clara. As I entered her room, she said with a smile, "The tests show you must be wrong. I just have a little blood problem."

Mark was looking at me expectantly; I had asked him to come so that we could all talk together.

I needed a minute to regroup my thoughts—all the preparation I had done before coming to her wasn't helping. Giving adverse news isn't new to an oncologist, but sometimes patients' overt optimism can throw you off balance.

"First let me see what's going on with your IV," I said. I took time checking her IV bag and the tubing that was running the fluid, and I gently touched her needle site. The nurse standing there was puzzled—she had just checked everything.

"You're right, Clara," I said, "you do have a blood problem."

"What kind?"

"I am afraid it's myeloma."

Her smile vanished and her face became dark. "Then it's like leukemia." She dissolved into tears, and her whole body shook. Mark was at a loss for a minute or two; then he sat on her bed and held her. I touched her shoulder to comfort her and waited. I tried to stay composed. After she settled down, I said, "I'll be back in the afternoon. We can talk about it then."

In the afternoon, she was calm and ready to know more. I explained myeloma in detail, including its treatment with melphalan, a chemo, along with prednisone, a mild steroid. Both were tablets and were taken in cycles: four to five days every five weeks. Melphalan, however, was the main drug and determined the treatment success, and prednisone alone wouldn't work.

"Once the protein and the calcium are reduced, you'll do well," I said to Clara.

I answered all the questions she and Mark had. "You need to sign a chemo consent form," I said. "The nurse will bring it to you."

Consent forms provide in writing what the patients need to know—what they are getting into. But the forms can be a double-edged sword. As a cancer doctor, in your discussion, you can temper your description; you emphasize the points that are more important than the others. You have to be measured without being misleading to keep the patient's hope alive, for hope is an important part of care. But consent forms have no room for discernment; all the possible complications in the book are listed, and even the mild ones look stark on paper. Cumulatively, this has a daunting effect on chemo patients. In truth, these forms are not just to inform but also to protect clinics, hospitals, and doctors from potential malpractice lawsuits.

When I returned later, Clara waved the form in front of me. "You expect me to sign this? The treatment can kill me."

"I believe I've gone through these things with you and Mark."

It has been well documented that cancer patients sometimes remember only part of the facts their doctors have given. It's shocking enough to find out you have cancer, and then the doctors and nurses are constantly throwing information at you. With all the mental pressure of the moment, your brain can absorb only so much.

On occasion, I had struggled to find a balance in bringing up serious matters to patients. I couldn't fault Clara for her reluctance to sign the form. Had

I failed in some way?

"Would you like a second opinion?" I asked. "I can send you to Houston."

"Not after what they did to my sister. The doctors acted like she wasn't all that important; they had too many patients like her."

"I know good doctors there."

"Are you trying to get rid of me?"

"No, but you have a choice."

Mark was glancing back and forth at his wife and me, as if he were searching for a solution.

"Do all the toxicities written here happen?" he asked me.

"Theoretically, yes. In practice, no." If I simply said yes, Clara could balk at chemo. Her kidney function was worsening, indicating that the M protein was increasing faster than before. She needed to start the treatment now before she was too sick to tolerate chemo. There's a point of no return in cancer, as in everything else in life.

I looked in Clara's eyes and said, "Remember, it's a partnership in fighting this cancer, a partnership between you and your family and me. You two talk some more and let me know." Then I left to finish my rounds.

After a few hours, the oncology nurse paged me and said, "Clara is ready for chemo." I gave the orders to start.

"Patient care is a joint decision," the ethicists rightly point out. But it's not always that simple. Ivory tower experts from a rarified atmosphere, with no bedside experience, often forget this: Each of us is our own person and lives life under our own circumstances, and we have our own hearts and minds. A uniform rule may not be useful to all.

I had seen West Texas farmers and ranchers with cancer, both men and women, who would say to me, "Talking too much isn't going to solve my problem. If something bad comes up, I can worry about it then. Do what you need to do now, Doc."

It's little different from my experience at Dhaka Medical College Hospital, except that the patients there were destitute and in a different culture and atmosphere. When I tried to explain complex treatments to them, some pleaded, "*Ami eshob bujhina, huzoor. Amar jiban Apnar hatey.* [I don't understand these things, sir. I put my life in your hands.]" What choice did the poor have but to put their lives on the line?

This unreserved confidence from patients, however, has another side with a perennial quandary. The stakes are raised, and things weigh on you more heavily. What if the treatment—especially chemo—ends up doing more harm than good?

Although melphalan isn't as harsh as some IV chemo drugs, it still has drawbacks. It invariably induces myelosuppression—suppression of the bone marrow (myelo means marrow)—leading to anemia and low white cells and platelets. Side effects are expected from all chemos in varying degrees—it's the nature of chemo. Problems arise if the cell counts drop to dangerous levels, and this is more likely in patients with organ dysfunction or debility. The consequences can be serious, including infections and bleeding. Fortunately, in the vast majority of patients, bone marrow and blood counts recover in time to safely begin the next chemo.

Clara tolerated the first treatment well. Her bone pain improved some after a few days, and she needed only a codeine combination, a low-tier narcotic, to control it. All this raised her spirits. Pain is always a demoralizing force, and its relief buoys patients.

There wasn't much else we could do except to let the chemo do its work. Hospitals are notorious for transmitting drug-resistant infections, so I discharged her. I would check her in the clinic in three weeks. Meanwhile, she would have weekly CBC—complete blood count—to measure the white cells, platelets, and hemoglobin (contained in the red cells). Periodic CBC would help me to find the nadir of her count, which, in turn, would help me to calibrate the doses of her future chemos. Oncologists aim for an equilibrium that controls the cancer while avoiding injury. I hoped that her myelosuppression, which would surely come, would be mild and that she wouldn't be susceptible to infection or bleeding.

I anxiously waited to see what would happen to her next.

I was relieved to see Clara's smile as I said hello to her in the clinic. In the three weeks since I had seen her, she had become a different person. Her spirits were higher and her bone pain was less than before. Her kidney function, too, had improved, and her calcium had become normal. This was a pleasant follow-up.

"I didn't go to my beautician, since you asked me not to," she said, "and I'm using a four-point walker at home."

I had advised her not to go out in public. With her immunosuppression, it would be easy to contract infection from others with coughs and colds. As for her walking, oncologists sometimes give seemingly conflicting advice, and I was no exception. Walking might be hazardous and cause her to fall and break her bones, then why recommend it? Because although she received pamidronate for her weak bones, it wasn't enough by itself. Ambulation (walking) also helps to build bones and heal lytic lesions. It also prevents thromboembolism—blood clots in the veins and lungs—that are serious threats to chronically bedridden patients.

"Do I have a good chance since I'm getting better?" Clara asked. "I miss my kids in school. I told you I wanted to go back to teaching."

Her optimism was a good sign. But she was asking me questions that I had already answered in the hospital. Again, it isn't unusual to forget what you heard under stress. Her prognosis remained very poor because she was at the highest stage of the disease. I hated to disabuse her of her new-found optimism, yet I felt an obligation not to sugarcoat what she was facing.

She heard me out and asked, "Am I doomed like my sister?"

"No, that's not what I was saying. You still have a chance. You're lucky, it's a treatable cancer."

"What luck," she said sarcastically. "Do you want that kind of luck for yourself?" Once more, the pitfalls of my unguarded words.

"I mean you can go into remission with chemotherapy."

But the term "remission" didn't satisfy her either. She asked me point blank, "Can you cure me?"

This was the question I was dreading, even though it's a routine one for practicing oncologists. Giving patients the harsh truth at the wrong time can lead to despair, and despair makes them forget the reasons to go on. So I offered what I thought was a milder answer.

"It's a difficult disease to cure, but some patients have lived for years with treatment."

The fact is that MM is an incurable cancer. Patients who have remission later relapse and die of the disease or its complications. At that time, the average life expectancy for Clara's kind of stage-three MM was two years, and hers was likely much shorter. (More recently, the outlook for myeloma has improved a lot.)

To encourage her, I also told her about a pertinent principle of cancer biology: each cancer in each person behaves in its own way. That's why patients sometimes do better than their doctors' predictions, regardless of the bad prognosis.

I had actually come to believe in this contradiction after running into a hard reality. Early in my practice, beginning in July 1975, my assiduous reading of the medical literature made me too confident about prognoses, and my pronouncements matched that. I was soon humbled by my limitations. In my training years in New York and Houston, on occasion, my distinguished teachers had also been wrong about outcomes. But medical technology and knowledge had advanced quickly since my training, with the arrival of CT and other new tests and treatments. I surmised things would be different now. Unfortunately, there wasn't enough of a difference. I can also look back and make a simple point: though new technology has improved patient care, it still can't supersede human judgment.

Like their patients, cancer doctors can't survive without optimism. I tried to find reasons to think optimistically of Clara's future. She was young, and apart from her kidneys, her vital organs—such as the heart, lungs, and liver— were functioning well. And she had made progress with the treatment.

Amid this good news came bad. Clara was readmitted to the hospital with a high fever and chills from an acute urinary tract infection. What I had been dreading about her bone marrow had happened. The chemotherapy had driven down her blood counts much lower than expected. And with her immunosuppressed state, infection and fever were dangerous. It was one of the medical emergencies in a cancer patient that had to be addressed quickly. Patients in Clara's state have died while waiting for the lab to confirm a diagnosis. Looking for immediate certainty is a fallacy here; there is no time to waste. You make the best clinical judgment possible and begin treatment, then modify it as you find out more.

Urinary tract infection is a common condition and is easily cured with oral antibiotics in otherwise healthy persons. But not in cases like hers. Her urine culture showed an infection by *Pseudomonas* bacteria, an aggressive organism. If the bacteria were to enter her bloodstream and induce sepsis, it could be lethal.

To make things worse, Clara's bacteria had shown resistance to all the antibiotics except one, gentamicin. The indiscriminate use of antibiotics had produced a pernicious effect, and more and more bacteria were becoming resistant to the common, safer antibiotics, curtailing their utility. As a society, we were paying a high price for our bad prescribing habits; hospitals everywhere were bedeviled by a super-bug called MRSA, methicillin-resistant *Staphylococcus aureus*.

Gentamicin would eradicate Clara's infection, but as usual, when it came to her, nothing was easy. Gentamicin is toxic to the kidneys and the inner ears, especially if its blood level exceeds the therapeutic level. The last thing she needed was kidney failure. Also troubling, the inner ear damage causes a side effect called vestibulopathy, which can induce imbalance and vision problems. If that happened, she would be prone to falling and crushing her bones.

Still, we had to take a chance, and as soon as possible. I told her about the difficulty we were facing. IV fluid and medications had brought her fever down. She had enough energy to argue back.

"What if my kidneys completely fail? In case you've missed it, they aren't healthy now either."

"I don't want that to happen. But if it does, we can take care of it with dialysis."

"No!" She was emphatic. "I know about dialysis. I don't want to live hooked up to machines and tubes."

"Dialysis, if needed, will be temporary," I reasoned. "Once the myeloma is controlled, your kidney function will come back. Dialysis has been successfully used in myeloma patients."

"I want to think about the antibiotic."

"We don't have time to wait. The antibiotic you're receiving now isn't working well. It's a bad infection, and we can't let the infection get the better of you."

She threw up her hands. "I knew you'd get your way."

We began gentamicin with caution and closely followed its blood level to regulate the dose, enough that it would work and yet keep the kidneys safe.

I was apprehensive about what I was doing to Clara. While I worried about possible unforeseen factors that could affect her systems, my assurance to her that dialysis would be temporary seemed shaky. I had no way of knowing that for sure. Dialysis would certainly complicate the course of her cancer. With her immunosuppression, it would increase the chances of "opportunistic infections." That term refers to an infection caused by the "friendly" or benign microbes that are normally present in our body. They do no harm to healthy persons but can turn ugly and attack seriously ill hosts; the microbes wait like the predators that pounce on the weakest animal. These infections are doubly hard to manage since the patients already have other burdens.

But if I didn't prescribe gentamicin, Clara was likely to die of sepsis. What good would the cancer therapy be then? I repelled my worries by recalling a distressing reality: my patients have to fight on multiple fronts, often at once, and my duty is to help them with the best defense at hand.

CHAPTER 2

L uck favored Clara. Her infection came under control and her fever subsided. I must admit that it wasn't due to the antibiotic alone. By then, her infection-fighting white cells had begun to increase. And the gentamicin had spared her kidneys.

But as happens with immunosuppressed patients, her troubles were far from over. How would she cope with her next round of chemo? Her cell counts weren't good enough to safely restart melphalan, which would inhibit them again. And melphalan, like most chemo, would bring on cumulative toxicities—that is, the more chemo you take, the more you weaken your marrow. Also, on rare occasions, melphalan can be spiteful, causing protracted myelosuppression. Therefore, adding more of it could be risky for patients like Clara. I couldn't forget, however, the crucial fact: whatever we did would matter little if the myeloma advanced—it was the cancer that would determine her fate.

I felt cornered like Clara. If the next chemo were delayed, the disease would overtake her body; but if we gave the drug during the suppression, we would be courting disaster. In the end, I decided to wait for the cell counts to improve, for in my mind, this was the safer path. Clara agreed. So, once she was well enough to function, she was sent home from the hospital.

Two weeks later, she was in my office for follow-up. She was physically stronger, but she wasn't the feisty woman I had known; she had become depressed and subdued.

Since her acute state had passed, I surmised that she had spent more time pondering her illness and thus had cause to be depressed. During her last hospitalization, she had pressed me again to talk about a cure. At last, in exasperation, I had sharply replied, "There isn't one." She didn't expect this bluntness, and I regretted my manner.

She always had questions for me in every encounter, but this time she remained silent. I empathized with her.

"It's not easy for you, Clara, I know," I said. "But if you give up, medicines won't do you any good."

"Why waste time trying?" she sighed.

"I don't think you mean what you're saying," I said. Then I reminded her what we had discussed when I began her treatment. "It's a partnership in fighting this cancer, a partnership between you and your family and me."

Clara burst into tears.

"What partnership?" she said through her tears. "It's been misery for me."

I handed her a tissue. She wiped her eyes and told me what was tormenting her besides the cancer.

"How can my own child do this to me?" she said. "Here I am dying, and she goes for this good-for-nothing boy. He'll ruin her life. I can't believe this is the girl I raised."

It was a kind of story that was familiar to me, and through time I had heard many variations of it from my patients. Nonetheless, it was distressing to see a mother in anguish.

This was about her older child, Tasha, who was nineteen. While we were talking, Eileen, my chemo nurse, knocked at the door. She never interrupted me unless there was an emergency. She needed to talk to me alone.

"A young woman has just shown up," Eileen said. "She's Clara's daughter, and she wants to see her mother right away. She got very angry when I asked her to wait. I'm afraid she's going to make a scene."

I respected Eileen's observations. I had been fortunate to work with nurses with a high level of discretion. Without their help, I wouldn't have succeeded. Nurses' insights help doctors care for patients; after all, it's routinely the case that nurses spend more time with patients than doctors do.

Clara also had a twelve-year-old son, Robby, whom I had met when he came before with his mother. At first, he was distraught seeing her suffer, but my reassurance and her improving health had put him at ease. I had not yet seen her daughter, and Clara hadn't previously spoken about their conflict. I went back to Clara and asked if Tasha could take part in our discussion.

"She's come out of guilt," Clara said. "Let her in."

Tasha didn't say hello to her mother or respond to my greeting when she entered the room. She stood quietly in a corner. I could see why a young man would fall for her. She was a lovely woman with pretty eyes and golden hair flowing down to her waist. It was obvious that she wasn't friendly like her brother and parents. She looked defiant. When I asked her if she had any questions, she said no and walked out of the room, slamming the door. I understood Clara's dejection.

Tasha was a student at Angelo State University. She had fallen in love with a classmate, Lance. Unfortunately, he was a drug addict. He wanted to be free of his addiction, he said, if Tasha would stand by him, and then they would make a future together. She felt sorry for him and bought into his promise.

But things didn't turn out the way they seemed when they began their friendship. Lance refused to go to rehab or meet with the school counselor. In the process of trying to change his behavior, Tasha became more and more entangled. After a while, like him, she started skipping classes. The situation only got worse: she took the tuition funds her parents had given her and dropped out of school without telling them. While Lance was sitting idle, she was working as a waitress to support them both.

"Can you believe this?" Clara said. "She has more sympathy for that addict than for me. And I'm her dying mother. I feel humiliated and helpless. She's mad because I was angry at her for not leaving that hopeless nobody. What should I live for? She's destroying my family. Her dad can't stand her anymore and they get into shouting matches. Poor Robby and I are caught in the middle."

I asked Clara if it would help if I discussed the gravity of her illness with Tasha.

"It won't do any good," she said. She was convinced that Tasha wouldn't care, whatever I told her.

Clara's feelings about Tasha echoed her feelings about chemo. She'd had enough of it. After I pleaded, however, Clara agreed to undergo the treatment again.

I wondered if I should get in touch with Tasha to talk. Yet, I was bound by the patient's privacy, and Clara hadn't given me permission.

A few days later, I got an unexpected call. It was Tasha.

"My mother must've told you how rotten I am and what an angel she is," she said. It was apparent that the mother and daughter had parallel feelings. Then she added, "But I'm not as bad as you think."

Should I reveal my patient's details to her? I reasoned that it would be better to do so, since Clara wasn't overtly opposed to the idea. I could use Tasha's overture to make some points that might benefit my patient. And perhaps it might also benefit the daughter.

"It's not that she thinks badly of you, Tasha," I said. "She worries about you and your future. All parents worry about their children. I worry about my children, too."

"I'm not a child anymore," she said. "Why can't my mother accept that I can run my own life? I don't want to be treated like dirt. Yes, my boyfriend isn't a saint. But he loves me, and I love him, and I'm helping him get over his addiction. Do you think her own husband is perfect? He drinks a lot, and rather than blaming him for that, she blames me." There was more to this hostility than I knew, but I had no desire to get drawn into the fray. It was better to say what I needed to say and leave it at that.

"Do you know how bad your mother's cancer is?" I asked. "You can help her recover."

"Yes, I've seen what she's been going through. But she won't take my help unless she gets her way. We've been fighting each other for a whole year, starting before her sickness. And now she's using her cancer as a gun to my head."

"It's unfair to say all that, Tasha."

"Not really," she bristled. "That woman is using the threat of her death to control me."

"You know better than that. Does your mother really want to die just to prove her point?"

There was silence. I waited. Then I heard a sob, and she began again.

"I don't want her to die. I hate her for what she does to me, but she's my mother. You wouldn't believe how close we used to be. There was a time when I could do nothing wrong, but now I can't do anything right."

Then she hung up.

It's an irony of life: betrayal by the ones you love the most is hardest to bear. In this case, each thought the other was betraying her.

Predictably, Clara had myelosuppression again after the latest chemo. Weeks went by, and her counts wouldn't budge. Cumulative toxicity was showing its malevolence, and I faced the same old quandary. If we waited too long, the myeloma would march on undeterred, and that would be the end of her. Still, I had no way of restarting the drug.

I searched for another agent that would be safe. Dr. Raymond Alexanian at the MD Anderson Cancer Center had a new treatment for myeloma: high-dose dexamethasone (dex), a stronger version of prednisone. This treatment had yet to become widely accepted, but I had great respect for Alexanian as a leader in myeloma research and therapy. Dex has one virtue that I sorely needed: it doesn't depress the bone marrow. It's also given orally in an off-and-on cycle.

I told Clara about dex.

"I'm glad you've found something that wouldn't hurt my blood," she said. "Why didn't you try it before?"

"We had to start with the standard chemo first."

"It couldn't be worse than melphalan."

She eagerly began taking dex. A few days later, she said, "It's a great medicine. I feel happy for the first time in a long time, and I'm eating better."

She was feeling the steroid's transient good effects: euphoria and increased appetite.

"My cancer must be doing better," she cheerfully added.

Indeed, after the first cycle of dex, her M protein level decreased.

"I told you it's working," she reminded me.

"We still have to watch out for toxicity," I cautioned her gently.

As time passed, Clara's disease got progressively better. For the first time, she complained about my exam room. "Can't you get rid of the drab carpet and put colorful pictures on the walls? It's not exactly a happy place—we don't come to see you for high blood pressure."

"I'll look into it," I said.

After about ten weeks, she gained weight, and her face became puffy and round; these changes seemed to happen unobtrusively. After another few weeks, though, her appearance was completely altered.

"Is this what you call helping?" she snapped at me. "Could I be any uglier than this? I hate looking in the mirror. I have no life." Then, pointing at her face and shoulders, she added, "What's the difference between living like this and dying of cancer?"

Dex, though not chemo, can be highly toxic in its own way—it spares the bone marrow at a cost. Clara was a victim of the insidious effects of the steroid, with fatty deposits on various parts of the body; her face was round like a full moon, and her shoulders had humps like a buffalo's. Moreover, dex had made her skin fragile, causing extensive bruises on the hands, legs, and abdomen, as if she had been beaten up.

What answer could I give to her question, "Is this what you call helping?"

Sure, dex was abating her cancer, but because of the side effects, I had no choice but to discontinue it. That's another paradox with which oncologists grapple—we are forced to abandon a treatment even if it's working because of its intolerable side effects.

What to do now? She could take neither chemo nor dexamethasone. Bone marrow transplant (BMT) is an option for MM, but it's a procedure fraught with complications that can be brutal.

I discussed the BMT option with Clara and Mark. Because she was only thirty-nine, I was willing to try this drastic procedure. But she flatly declined.

"I don't want to suffer from treatments anymore," she said.

After a while, she complained that her bones were hurting again. Without any treatment, her cancer was gaining the upper hand. Soon, her life became hellish from the ferocious pain.

Strong narcotics made Clara's life livable. But depression overcame her psyche, and counseling was of little help. She thought her death wasn't far off. She worried about her husband and son, and she was torn about her daughter. Clara did a lot of soul searching.

"Mark and Robby will manage somehow," she said, "but Tasha will be ruined. Who'll save her from her own madness?"

Her daughter became her obsession. I asked Mark for that Ann Landers remedy, family counseling—at least, the mother and the daughter together. I made it clear that they didn't have much time to lose; they must reconcile now or never.

"You're telling me something that I've tried," he said. "At one time, those two women couldn't be separated. But now, they won't even talk to each other. I need to watch my boy and my wife and not worry about Tasha."

Clara's condition warranted my placing her in hospice. "Hospice can make your days easier," I said to her, "and they're good at controlling pain." I went through all the details of hospice and added, "I strongly recommend it."

But she hesitated. Though the first hospice in the US, Connecticut Hospice, was started in 1974, the program was still misunderstood by many. Some believed it to be a "death house," as did Clara. This perception came from the fact that most patients died within six months of entering its service. But that was simply because they were terminal—destined to die, hospice or not.

I had been the voluntary medical director of an emerging nonprofit hospice in our community, and I urged Clara to at least talk to one of its nurses. "If you don't like what they do, you're free to refuse," I reassured her.

She agreed to meet with a nurse. In general, human beings are willing to accept death, but we dread the agony of pain.

A hospice nurse patiently gave Clara time and attention and was able to allay her fears and reservations. Clara could stay at her home among her loved ones, and the caregivers would check her routinely and adjust her medications, particularly the narcotics. In addition, they would always be on hand, day or night, weekday or weekend—just a phone call away.

In the end, Clara consented. For her, hospice was indeed a godsend. High doses of morphine, combined with antianxiety medications, changed her outlook. She began to show more interest in living.

Cancer is just one hardship for the terminally ill. Unfortunately, treatment of the symptoms can engender more of the same. Narcotics cause constipation and nausea and can make a person drowsy and confused. All this can unsettle patients and their loved ones. Hence, empathy and patience are essential in caring for the dying, but these alone aren't enough. Loneliness often becomes an enemy, and patients feel abandoned. The living may not notice any of these changes, immersed as they are in running their own lives. Not surprisingly, Clara couldn't escape these challenges. What brought light and hope to her were the interest and kindness of the hospice professionals.

I asked our hospice to make an exception for Clara. They would perform a CBC every so often to see whether her blood count had improved. I was still hoping to try more of the melphalan, however remote the chance. Hospices are reimbursed by Medicare and must follow its rules, which only allow palliative measures. Aiming for remission was out of the question. But I argued that melphalan might keep the myeloma at bay and lessen the pain, thereby improving Clara's quality of life. In that sense, melphalan, though a chemo, was palliative for her. Of course, I wanted to prolong her life if I could do so safely, but I kept that thought to myself.

Some patients, in their final days, face immense physical and mental anguish. Right or wrong, by now, I had learned to bend the rules a bit for their sake. But even for hospice, cost is a factor, and medicines are costly. I had to justify the cost.

"If we can reduce or stop some of the medications by giving melphalan," I argued, "it'll save money. And it's only a tablet, not an IV injection, and inexpensive as chemo goes."

I also found a reason to do her blood counts.

"If her anemia gets worse, she'll be weaker and more anorectic, and a simple blood transfusion will make her stronger. She'll be able to take more food and fluid. After all, the motto of hospice is to make life easier for patients, is it not?"

For good reasons, hospices don't do tests just to satisfy the curiosity of doctors and families. But when a patient suddenly gasps for air or has wild hallucinations, their loved ones, in desperation, may ask, "Why don't you do some x-rays and labs to find out what's going on?"

What's going on, of course, is that the cruel cancer is having its way. Invasive tests are of no use for the patients' welfare; besides, some tests are painful. A few hospices, however, avoid necessary tests or medicines simply because of the payment system. Hospices receive a fixed reimbursement for each patient, and since tests and medicines cut into the revenue, they lower the profit. A few for-profit hospices have used the abhorrent practice of cutting corners at the expense of the terminally ill. When they are caught by Medicare, they are penalized. But rogue hospices are rare exceptions. Overall, the benefits of hospice are obvious: the dying no longer have to stay in the hospital to die; they can spend their remaining days at home with their families. Moreover, hospices are far less expensive than hospitals.

I was willing to assist Clara in any way possible. But once she became stable, I mostly left it to the hospice to manage her palliation. I had too many other patients needing my time. Clara understood that. In any hospice, doctors are a part of the team, but it's the nurses, social workers, pastoral counselors, and volunteers who give daily medical, emotional, and spiritual support to the terminally ill.

I talked to Clara by phone off and on, and there were times when she hardly made sense because of the narcotics. Mark's appraisal was usually something like, "She's hanging in there as best she can."

Three months into hospice care, a nurse informed me that Clara's blood counts had gone up.

"She's ready to try melphalan if you are. I've talked to both her husband and her when she's alert, and they feel she's up to it now."

I had eagerly awaited this news. But now that it had come, I wavered. I kept wondering if the repeat chemo would bring back her infections, since her blood counts would surely drop, and I had no way of knowing how much. I did know, however, what melphalan had done to her before.

My heart said to give it a try. She was young, with a family. Maybe we could fend off death for a while. My mind warned that it might be a mistake, with all those incalculable risks. Selfish thoughts also encroached on my thinking: Don't you remember how time-consuming she had been? And do you want to get into her family mess, and hear the endless complaints about her daughter? Right now, the hospice is handling all this, and she's taking little of your time. Staying out of their way is the prudent option. She will easily accept your decision of no further chemo.

On such occasions, logic is of no use to cancer doctors, because uncertainty is a regular part of our work. In this case, the heart won out. First, I went to see Clara at her home. We all put our brains together and concluded that melphalan was worth a retry. But Clara, being Clara, added a condition.

"You can only stick me every two months for the blood counts, that's all. I'm tired of the needles."

This was not how chemo was practiced. I would have no way of knowing the nadir of her counts. Besides the risks, how would I determine the next dose of melphalan if she was lucky enough to get it again?

She had no interest in my reasoning, however.

"Look, you've explained this mumbo-jumbo too many times," she said. "I'm the one who's taking the risks. This cancer is going to get me sooner or later—that's what I've understood from all of you doctors. The treatment gives me some hope. I'm not as callous as I might seem."

Fair enough. She had her own logic, which I couldn't dispute. But now the hard part. What dose to give? The textbook advice is to give the optimum dose. In oncology, that basically means to give as much as the patient's systems can tolerate. Biologically, this makes sense. Too low a dose to avoid side effects has its own hazard: it will not be enough to kill the cancer cells, which will then find ways to develop resistance. And there are hard facts to consider. Even with the maximum tolerable dose, drug resistance is a common curse with cancer treatment and is the primary cause of cancer deaths. Those malignant cells are extremely cunning—while you are giving chemotherapy, they are silently mutating to change their character and learning how to circumvent the chemical onslaught. This is akin to what bacteria, fungi, and viruses do as they develop resistance to antibiotics.

Going through all these mental exercises was fine in theory, but I still had to decide on her dose. What options did I have except to exercise my best judgment? Was I using the term "judgment" to hide my best guess? In any case, I calculated an amount that I thought was proper in her state of health. If my judgment turned out to be sound, she would be safe. If not, she would again be in acute peril, and I would bring her closer to death.

I anxiously waited after the first dose to see what would happen. Though I was concerned about Clara's blood counts, I kept my part of the bargain and didn't order the CBC during the interval. Luck saved us one more time—nothing unexpected happened. In two months, her counts were in an acceptable range.

Since there was no needle involved, Clara had no objection to collecting her urine. The result was more than gratifying—her M protein was lower than before.

She was willing to continue the chemo since she was getting better and stronger. So, I gave her another course. I wasn't going by the book, and I chose a dose based on my intuition.

Clara's days were good and bad, though more of the former now. Pain was still a concern, but less so than before, and we slowly lowered the amount of morphine. She was well enough to come to my clinic for follow-ups. Her hospice nurses were willing to bring her to me if her husband was busy at work. They had noticed how much the treatment had helped her.

Clara, however, didn't want to make the trip to the clinic.

"What's the purpose of my going to you just for a melphalan prescription?"

"I need to carefully examine you first," I said, "before I can give you more chemo."

But she wouldn't agree with me, and we were at a stalemate.

CHAPTER 3

C lara wouldn't break the stalemate; she wanted her way. She insisted on staying at home and continuing the melphalan plan. What could we do except to give in to her? Months passed in a blur, and she became more active. Hospices can only accept patients whose life expectancy is six months or less. This discourages abuse of the system. Without such limits, they could admit all kinds of non-terminal, chronically ill patients—and there are millions of them—to fatten their purses. And indeed, some hospices did so until they were discovered and punished. But the law also knows that doctors are not gods, even though some of them act like they are. Their estimates are just that—estimates—and patients may survive longer than six months. To accommodate these quirks, the rules allow the patients to stay in hospice, but with a condition: their doctors must certify the need to continue.

I certified Clara after checking her and consulting her nurses.

As her pain diminished in intensity, her morphine dose was cut again. By then, her moon face and buffalo humps had resolved a lot, and with that, her future outlook brightened.

At the time, I had no idea how her lytic lesions were faring. I hadn't given her the monthly IV pamidronate, the bone-healing medication, which she had gotten in the hospital; that would have been too much to ask without flouting the rules. But I knew that her increased activity would be helping her bones. Besides, the control of myeloma may have hardened her skeleton. The reduction in her bone pain supported these assumptions.

Another six months passed by in a flash. And a whole year had gone by since I fell into her orbit. I was happy that she had defied our predictions. Be that as it may, to maintain the hospice care, I had to again endorse its need. But the question that she and I had avoided so far couldn't be avoided now.

Since she was functioning fairly well, could she and her family manage by themselves? Both the hospice and I brought up the matter with her.

She made it clear that she was afraid to let go of the hospice, and, uncharacteristically, she begged me to agree.

"They've changed my life," she said. "I wouldn't be here without their care at home. To tell you the truth, I would've died if you had kept me in the hospital." And as if to entice me, she added, "I'll take the chemo as long as you want, and you can do your tests whenever you need."

She was, of course, right about the value of hospice. It allowed her to stay at her own place, surrounded by family and friends, in peace, without the tumult of a hospital. And she had developed close friendships with the nurses, social workers, and counselors. This intimacy had also fueled her desire to live. The main question became: would she deteriorate without hospice? I wasn't sure, but I shared her fear, so again I set out to accommodate her wish. But I couldn't do so without a reason.

Anyone who had beaten such unbelievable odds as hers deserved an unusual chance. But was this a good enough reason? Not really, for rules don't consider your feelings. Still, I signed her paperwork again, saying what was plausible: to sustain the quality of her life, she needed to continue hospice care.

I immediately felt conflicting emotions after I entered my signature. Was I subverting regulations because of my bond with Clara? Was I breaching any ethics? I couldn't escape the weight of my responsibility: I was her physician as well as the hospice medical director—the onus fell squarely on me.

I felt justified that granting her the relief she had requested was the right thing to do. Besides, if she ended up in the hospital, the cost of her care would certainly be higher, with her insurance and Medicare having to fork out huge sums of money.

Looking back on Clara's ordeal, I was amazed at her resilience, as were the hospice staff. Witnessing suffering and death is the inescapable lot of oncologists, and stories like Clara's soften our heartache and grief. They also make doctors humble and receptive. I remember a surgeon's remark about Clara when I asked him to put in an indwelling IV catheter. This happened at the time when she came to the hospital with fever and infection, and she needed the catheter quickly to get antibiotics and fluids. My surgical colleague was busy, and he didn't share my sense of urgency.

"Can't you wait a little?" he asked. "If you look at her whole picture, what difference will we make?"

After Clara's one year was over, I made a point of updating that surgeon about her status—how she had turned around. "My God!" he said. "I can't believe it. Reading her records, I didn't think she could last long. I see that my conclusion was wrong."

Clara's second extension with hospice, like the first, seemed to finish too soon. She was inching closer to normal. She was still reluctant to part with the hospice care, which brought us face-to-face with the recurring tension. The hospice nurses got nowhere by pleading that the need for their services had passed. The bond between Clara and me began to strain again.

I went to her home to talk. She greeted me warmly and asked me to sit at her dining table. Then she went to get me a cup of tea—she knew I enjoyed hot tea. While waiting, I looked through a window. It was a bright afternoon, and birds were singing in the oaks—songbirds always made me happy. She had birdfeeders outside the window, and several white-wings were jostling each other and eating the seeds. I was surprised to see them; they were mostly South Texas doves that had begun to migrate to West Texas. There was a garden next to a glass panel, where a pair of hummingbirds fluttered for nectar. Their feathers flashed in a beam of sunlight as they zoomed back and forth, proving that hummingbirds are the only birds that can fly forward and backward and hover. A thought crossed my mind: why was I here to spoil a day like this for Clara and me?

"They're lovely, don't you think?" Clara startled me. I hadn't heard her light footsteps. "They sure are," I replied.

She put the cup on the table and pulled up a chair in front of me. I glanced at her as I drank. It dawned on me that I had been so preoccupied with relieving her illness that I had forgotten the person herself. Her moon face and buffalo humps were almost gone, and most of her old glow had returned. With her combed hair—she had little hair loss from the melphalan—and stylish blouse and skirt, she looked beautiful. And she moved around easily

41

before she sat. She thanked me for coming to check on her, and there was a wide smile on her face.

After a few pleasantries, I forced myself to delve into the heart of the issue. Otherwise, I was afraid I might leave without fulfilling my intended obligation.

"We can't ignore the rules at will, Clara," I said. "We need to cut off the hospice; you're doing well."

"I don't care about your rules," she retorted, her arms folded defiantly. "I'm alive because of them, am I not?" Her face stiffened, her smile fading.

We were at a stalemate again. "We'll discuss it another time with Mark and you together," I said and got up to leave.

"I can decide for myself. Mark has enough on his shoulders. He works long hours; we have bills to pay."

Although many people are a part of a hospice team, the nurses carry the lion's share of the burden. A few days later, the nurse who was closely involved with Clara called me. She sounded frustrated as well. And believe me, these nurses don't get frustrated easily.

"Clara wants to go to her weekly beauty shop appointments," the nurse said. "And she's eating and drinking regularly. She can do without morphine now. We've tried to slowly withdraw the morphine and try a codeine combination. But she insists on keeping her old routine. We don't know what to do."

I sympathized with the nurse. I wanted to talk to Clara again to settle the matter, but this time in my office, in case we ran into another argument. When my assistant called her to schedule an appointment, Clara was indignant. She wouldn't go out and sit in the clinic, she said, when she wasn't looking her best.

It's a good sign when patients are interested in self-care and grooming, because it means they are interested in life. But as good as all that was, I had to put my foot down. In the interest of her welfare, I had been willing to *bend* a few rules, but I wasn't willing to *break* them to satisfy her whims. I remembered my old days, when most of the patients died in hospitals, amid the restrictive and sterile atmosphere. And how hospices had become the refuge for the dying. I was moved to promote their cause by writing a widely read article for the *Wall Street Journal* (November 2, 1995). How could I be a part of getting a hospice in trouble just for Clara?

I found no justification to accommodate Clara any longer. I firmly told her that I would refuse her hospice extension unless she came for a checkup.

She grudgingly made an appointment with me. I did the essential myeloma tests. To my pleasant surprise, her M protein was gone, and her kidneys were near normal. And her blood counts showed significant progress, as did the x-rays of her bones. She had responded to melphalan.

I was one thankful oncologist.

When I gave her the news, her attitude instantly changed. She became less confrontational, and without protest, she even agreed to a bone marrow aspiration and biopsy.

I should have guessed the marrow result before the test—the plasma cells had followed the rest; they were also normal. She had no evidence of myeloma. Finally, we were able to release her from hospice without friction.

Oncologists don't have simple vocabularies for their diagnoses or drugs; the terms tend to be long and complex. Sometimes it isn't easy to convey the concepts to patients and others. Even non-oncologist physicians complain about this. But that doesn't mean cancer doctors don't like ordinary words. They do, and there are two plain words they dearly cherish: "complete remission." Or, in oncology parlance, CR. Happily, Clara was in CR.

The CR would have been a celebration for all, but there was a new rub— she had become addicted to morphine.

It's not that I didn't worry about addiction. But when you have terminal cancer and horrendous pain, and the narcotics give you the relief and motivation to go on living, the last thing you worry about is what's in the future, including the potential for addiction, because there's no future to think of.

Cancer pain creates a vicious circle: uncontrolled pain demoralizes patients and magnifies the severity of their physical and psychological woes. Again, I couldn't help remembering my student and training years in Dhaka and the US. Because of the fear surrounding narcotics, they were avoided or given in inadequate doses, and I witnessed how cancer patients went through uncalled-for agony, even at academic centers. And my experience with Tobi, the nine-year-old boy with sarcoma at Dhaka Medical College Hospital, still haunted me at times. It was the same way when I began my practice in 1975. In time, seeing the persistent attitude, I made an impassioned plea on behalf of patients called "Narcotics for Cancer Patients," in the *New York Times* (June 12, 1987): "Of course, narcotics are serious drugs. They should be administered for only one reason—to control disabling pain. We should try to understand the difficulties of patients with incurable cancer, their anguish and despair, and strive to enhance the quality of their lives."

I used my own counsel on Clara. But cancer, being capricious, creates unforeseen calamities. While you are intensely absorbed in the crisis of the present, another enemy covertly creeps up on you. Then you end up courting an unintended sorrow. As a patient, you have a ready defense—you got addicted to a drug that was prescribed to you. You were merely following directives.

The current opioid crisis, however, is a tragedy of an entirely different kind; it's the result of indiscriminate prescribing and outright drug abuse. To bring a balance to pain medicine prescription, medical organizations such as the American Society of Clinical Oncology (ASCO), to which I belong, have issued guidelines on pain management. But the guidelines alone aren't a solution to such an important issue for medicine and the public. How did it come to this? How did we go from underprescribing to overprescribing opioids? Again, it's because of our lack of knowledge of opioids and our thoughtlessness about chronic pain control. Bioethicist Travis Rieder of Johns Hopkins, himself a victim of both underprescribing and overprescribing, pointed to the core of the problem in a 2019 *Nature* essay: "Pain education is often an afterthought in medical schools; many medical students graduate without taking any courses on pain."

I don't disavow my basic premise written for the *New York Times* thirty-seven years ago—the need to use enough narcotics to relieve devastating pain caused by refractory cancer. To be sure, narcotic addiction is rare in cancer pain treatment, because almost all patients stop the drug once the cancer is controlled.

Whatever the merits of my philosophy, I couldn't turn back the clock on Clara, and I had to deal with the difficulty at hand.

"You need to get off morphine completely," I said to her. "This will give you more freedom."

"Don't lecture me on this," she said. "The nurses have already told me enough."

For addicts, addiction is a sensitive subject.

"I'll give you something else for your pain," I said, "something that's less harmful."

"Have you been sleepless night after night?" she said. "Morphine helps me to sleep well. If you take it away, I'll die of insomnia. The cancer is going to come back anyway. You haven't mentioned a cure."

"Let's stick to the point. You know morphine isn't a sleeping pill."

"For me, it is."

"I'll give you methadone to handle the withdrawal," I reassured her. "If anyone can fight an addiction, you can. You've already cut down the doses before. And you've beaten an almost fatal cancer. Remember, your constipation and nausea will go away if you get rid of morphine, and you won't need the medications for them."

"If you're that concerned about morphine, why did you give it to me in the first place?"

"You know why."

Despite her grumbling, she gave it a try, and after several weeks, she became free of the narcotic. In retrospect, she was more habituated than addicted. There are disputes concerning how to define habituation versus addiction. A simple question may distinguish the two: can the person function normally without the substance? In habituation, skipping or stopping the drug may cause mild psychological effects: for example, irritation, restlessness, insomnia, or a feeling of missing something. Addiction is entirely different. Withdrawing the substance will cause severe physical and psychological havoc.

Alcoholism, which seems more socially acceptable than drug abuse, illustrates addiction. The sudden withdrawal of alcohol results in delirium tremens (DT); patients develop mental confusion and severe autonomic hyperactivity, which may lead to cardiovascular collapse. Hence, DT is a medical emergency, and without prompt treatment, it has a high rate of fatality.

"I admire your pluck," I said to Clara in the course of one of our conversations.

"I've given you a lot of headaches and worries," she replied, "but I want you to know you're special."

I hadn't been quite sure how she had felt about me, with all our arguments and conflicts. Worse, I had given her a death sentence before its time. It's strange that our outer manner may not reflect our inner feelings—antagonism can mask friendship or friendship, hostility.

Clara came for follow-ups at quarterly intervals. I was pleased with how she was doing. After three years, however, things began to change. She became irregular with her visits to my office.

A year or so later, she stopped coming altogether. I called her and made a compromise. Sometimes compromise is in the nature of cancer practice. Since any doctor could order the protein studies, she could get them done by her family physician, who could then send the reports to me. She kept her promise only for some time, and then, inexplicably, she stopped seeing both her family physician and me.

Time passed, and Clara came to my mind less and less often. One day, I happened to come across a man who was our mutual acquaintance. He immediately evoked Clara's memory in me. When I asked him about her, he said that a friend had told him she had died a short while before. I felt a pang in my heart. But when I looked at her medical records, I felt comforted. She had lived for twelve years after her diagnosis, when her expected survival was two years at best.

Life went on as it always does, and as the years accumulated, Clara slipped out of my mind.

CHAPTER 4

It was one of my hectic days in the hospital, and I was preoccupied with a few acutely ill patients. As I was leaving the ward, Trish, the head nurse in oncology, picked up a page for me. "You've got a consult on a dialysis patient," she said. "She insists on seeing you as soon as possible. I think you should stop by her room."

I would rather have come back later to see the referral. Practicing oncologists often face time predicaments. When you go to a patient's room, you can't simply say to her or him, "This is the cancer and this is the treatment," then walk away. You have to connect: discuss the nature of the cancer, its prognosis, treatment options and their benefits and side effects, and then answer questions. But since one question inevitably leads to another, it can be time-consuming.

But Trish, like Eileen, my oncology nurse at the office, was a perceptive observer and had reasons for her suggestions. I walked to the patient's room, and at her door, I stopped in my tracks. She noticed my expression.

"What's the matter, Dr. R?" she said. "You look like you've seen a ghost."

"I didn't expect to see *you* here," I gushed.

"Well, some other Clara Anderson died, and I got the blame for it. Everybody knows I was supposed to die a long time ago."

It had been sixteen years since her diagnosis! And four years since the news of her "death."

She had been admitted to the hospital for unremitting diarrhea from an intestinal infection. And as she had done before, she agreed to go to the ER only when forced by her illness. She had lost so much fluid that she became badly dehydrated and went into acute renal failure. To save her life, she was put on dialysis, the very procedure that she had detested.

"Dr. Stevens says I have protein in the urine," Clara informed me, "and he's checking to see why."

"You know, Clara," I reassured her, "some infections can bring on abnormal proteins in the urine, and they go away when the infections are gone. I wouldn't worry."

"But this is complete kidney shutdown; how can I not worry?"

"Your kidneys were weak to start with and now this dehydration made it worse. It's temporary."

What I said about infection and that much dehydration was true. But she, being a cancer veteran, read right through me. Perhaps I was reassuring myself rather than her. Though she was clearly concerned about possible recurrence, her attitude had changed. She was more at ease with herself. Hearing her story, I couldn't disagree with her; she was, once again, in a precarious state. Why did it have to be her? I suppressed my feelings of foreboding.

"Give me a little time, we'll figure things out," I said and left to return later.

Clara's nephrologist gave me a rundown on her course in the hospital. When I asked him how he had convinced her to accept the dialysis, he said, "She had little choice—either do dialysis or die."

I reviewed her current records, labs, and x-rays, and compared them with what she had before. I found what I prayed not to find. The same M protein, the myeloma protein, had reappeared in her urine and in a much larger quantity. This was blocking her kidneys as it had done the first time, except now with acute dehydration, her kidneys had completely failed. Her present disease was most likely fatal.

Oncologists are sometimes confounded when patients in CR for a long time get cancer again; this baffles the patients, too. Is this a relapse or an entirely new primary malignancy? In Clara's case, the M protein turned out to be identical, so it was a recurrence.

"Where was my cancer all these years?" Clara asked me. "You said I had complete remission. Then how could I have the same myeloma again?"

I decided to use basic oncologic biology to explain the recurrence of her cancer, rather than just saying that a plasma cell mutates to become malignant.

We have special cells in our body called stem cells, which are the parent cells that produce each of our organs and tissues, such as the heart, lungs, liver, kidneys, brain, and bone marrow. Somehow, one of the parent cells turns malignant and multiplies endlessly, breaking the rules of the normal control. This unchecked proliferation is cancer. When patients receive chemo, some malignant stem cells evade the drugs and hide in the patients' systems, and we can't detect them with our tests. They silently reproduce more of their kind and, in the end, show up as recurrence. All this may take anywhere from weeks to years, and in some cases, even decades.

"CR and cure aren't the same thing, Clara," I said. "That's why you may remember I cautioned you about possible relapse."

"I didn't want to think about relapse back then. What's my prognosis this time?"

"Once a cancer recurs, the chance of its remission goes down. And with each recurrence, it finds new ways to become more resistant. This is the nature of cancer."

She didn't seem to be perturbed by my answer and said, "That's true if I go by the book, correct?"

"Yes."

Now she turned the tables on me.

"But I haven't gone by the book—you've said that many times. You see, now I need to defy the book even more than before."

"What're you getting at?"

"My son has two little boys, and they're very attached to their grandma. They think I hung the moon. I need to be around for them."

I remembered her son, Robby, a gentle boy of twelve. He was a man now, a father and a great comfort to his mother.

Grandchildren can be a powerful influence. We may not oblige others in the family, but we oblige our grandchildren. Patients may even accept treatment to stay alive if only because they want to see their grandchildren graduate or attain some other milestone.

"My grandson is getting married in a month," a hopelessly ill grandmother once told me. "He wants me to be at his wedding. He loves me so much, I'll do anything I can not to disappoint him." She died shortly after the wedding.

I saw many more examples like this over the years. A diehard scientist may dismiss these happenings as chance events, but I can't—medicine is full of mystery.

When I went back to Clara to talk about her treatment plan, a young woman was sitting at her bedside. Seeing me, the stranger promptly said, "I'm Tasha, Dr. Rahman."

My face must have shown surprise. She laughed and said, "Don't you remember that angry girl?"

"We couldn't have done without Tasha," Clara broke in. "She helps us a lot. She's a blessing. Mark's oil field work isn't going well."

Sixteen years had done something to this young woman. She was now poised and gentle. She had become a manager of a big department store. Past scenes crowded my mind—her hatred for her mother, her fights with her father, our tense encounter in my office, and our conversation on the phone. All this had been due to a drug-addicted boyfriend. What had happened to that boy? Had she turned him around as she had done for herself? But I checked my curiosity—neither the mother nor the daughter mentioned his name.

"What about my mom's treatment?" Tasha asked.

"We have a new kind of myeloma drug called Velcade. It's not like the regular chemo drugs. It's easier than chemo, and it doesn't damage the kidneys or white cells."

I needed to bring up another matter with Clara, and I had an idea of how she would react. "The combination of IV Velcade and oral dex is more effective than Velcade alone."

"Don't mention that steroid again," she snapped.

"We should take advantage of all the benefits we can get. The dex dose is lower now, and the lower dose is less toxic. We have to tackle the myeloma as soon as possible. Don't you want to get off dialysis?"

"You always put me in a tough spot."

Tasha, the once-impatient girl, now showed remarkable composure. She took the whole discussion in stride and addressed her mother, "I'm with Dr. Rahman, Mom."

Clara agreed to the drug combination. After a while, her kidneys recovered enough to stop dialysis. As usual, she appeared to be full of miracles. She achieved complete remission again, with normal bone marrow and normal M protein, the kind of outcome oncologists long for.

Clara's new CR didn't take away my perpetual worry. One relapse tends to portend another. Though she had had a long remission, this time the disease had progressed much more quickly. So, to consolidate a CR like this, adjuvant BMT was an option. The idea was to extend the CR as long as possible. Bone marrow transplant isn't a cakewalk, though some of its proponents have portrayed it so. In reality, it's fraught with danger.

Still, for hematologic cancers like myeloma, leukemia, and lymphoma, high-dose chemo with BMT made biological sense. The combination had worked in my leukemia and lymphoma patients, but when it came to myeloma, I couldn't get rid of my hesitation about transplant. Several of my myeloma patients had been luckless with BMT; they had relapsed and died after a short while. The procedure, however, was regularly used at the top cancer centers, and BMT was still an accepted choice for MM.

"We need to do something to prevent another relapse," I said to Clara.

"Do you always have to mention relapse?" she protested.

"That's the nature of things, and you're only fifty-five. We should do BMT."

"I've read about BMT. It sounds good, if that's what you want."

Because BMT had worked in blood cancers, quite a few experts promoted it for common tumors like breast, without solid evidence. Its apparent success in this malignancy was coming out more and more in magazines and newspapers, and its devastations were glossed over. A bandwagon effect took over the transplant concept. Breast cancer, unlike hematologic cancers, is so widespread that BMT became a profitable business for big hospitals, both academic and private. Desperate breast cancer patients were taken advantage of with flimsy promises. I was particularly saddened by the horrifying end of a few of these women. Not surprisingly, the breast-BMT business became scandal-plagued when an outright fraud was discovered in a transplant study; the study's positive result had been fabricated by one of its physician researchers. Subsequently, breast-BMT died its deserved death due to its futility, but only after wreaking havoc on many lives.

As it turned out, Clara had read several of these glossed-over articles. She had forgotten that we had discussed the transplant when we stopped the melphalan. She had declined it at the time because of its risks. I couldn't blame her memory; sixteen years is a long time, and she was so sick at the time. I had an advantage—I had her medical records to remind me.

So, when she said the transplant "sounds good," I had to caution her. "I'm afraid BMT isn't that trouble-free. It has big hazards."

Clara was vexed. "I've just begun to taste normal life again," she groaned. Then she curtly added, "Leave me alone."

Realizing how she had just acted, she tried to soften her remark.

"If you were doing the transplant yourself, I might've agreed. But you're trying to send me to a big cancer center. I don't want to be a number."

She was right on both counts. Although I was practicing in good hospitals, we had a relatively small number of transplant candidates, so we couldn't justify having a BMT program. A large referral center that does a complex procedure every day will do it better than a center that does it occasionally. That's why we sent our transplant patients to the programs in Houston, Dallas, or San Antonio. Some of my patients had complained to me about the impersonal bedside manner of a few of the big-city doctors.

Clara looked me straight in the eyes and asked, "If you were me, would you invite misery when you're feeling good?"

It's a question that many others had asked me. Patients want to know what I would do if I were them. Or, a patient's loved ones may ask, "What if she were your mother? What choice would you make?"

The trouble is that in cancer care, individuals do what they do according to the circumstances they find themselves in. Some decisions are clear-cut, and some are not. It's the gray areas that spawn ethical dilemmas. Clara's question, therefore, wasn't rhetorical; indeed, it had both ethical and practical implications when it came to BMT and myeloma. To complicate the decision, I had recently learned that new drugs for the disease were about to come onto the market.

I answered Clara, "For myself, I'm not sure what I'd do about BMT, but I know I'd get a second opinion from a BMT center before making my decision."

"Don't you think the BMT doctors would be biased in favor of BMT?"

"Some aren't biased."

"You don't want to carry my burden all by yourself, right?"

"Yes."

Clara and I discussed various BMT centers in Texas, including the University of Texas Southwestern Medical Center in Dallas, Methodist Hospital in San Antonio, and MD Anderson Cancer Center in Houston. But Texas is huge, and these places are 200 to 400 miles from San Angelo— long distances for anyone seeking treatment, and doubly hard for the sick and the weak.

I had mainly worked with two accomplished BMT doctors: Fred LeMaistre in San Antonio and Bob Collins in Dallas. Though I knew many of the oncologists at MD Anderson well—including Gabriel Hortobagyi, a leader in the breast cancer field; Hagop Kantarjian, a leukemia pioneer; and Nizar Tannir, a force in urologic oncology—I had no good connection with its BMT department.

Clara chose San Antonio because it was the closest of the three cities. I had been referring patients to Fred LeMaistre and his colleague, Carlos Bachier, also a top clinician, for quite a few years. I also had a personal reason for recommending Fred. His late father, Charles LeMaistre, was a past president of MD Anderson Cancer Center for many years, and he was kind to me. Moreover, at different periods, Fred's father and I served as trustees of Austin College, a first-rate liberal arts college in Sherman, Texas.

Carlos and Fred examined Clara. Their conclusion was what I had expected. She was a suitable transplant candidate because of her history—one relapse already, a relatively young age, and current good physical condition. Besides, the BMT complications would likely be more tolerable at this time than if she recurred again.

I trusted Carlos and Fred, and Bob Collins in Dallas. It's well known that trust between patients and doctors is essential for good medical care; less well known is that trust among treating physicians is also important for patients' welfare. I also liked something else about these specialists: they didn't have the academic snobbery of some others I knew and were sympathetic to the difficulties of community oncologists.

BMT is inherently hazardous because of the nature of the procedure. You first give high-dose chemo to ostensibly eradicate all the cancer. In the process, the normal blood cells are also completely wiped out. In other words, the patient develops severe and prolonged myelosuppression, worse than with standard chemo.

After the chemo is done, you infuse the bone marrow of a healthy, matched donor into the patient. Through the circulation, the stem cells from the donor's marrow will travel to the recipient's marrow bed and settle there, then generate normal white cells, red cells, and platelets. It takes weeks for the new marrow to be active. In the intervening period, the patient is defenseless against dangerous infections.[1]

After Clara got the BMT opinion, she said, "I need to have *some* good time with my grandchildren. For the first time in their lives, I'm able to do things with them." Then she implored, "Am I wrong if I don't do the transplant now?"

I wished I had oracular powers. I didn't know what to say. My silence must have sent a dispiriting message, and she appeared lost.

Looking at her downcast face, I said, "If you want to wait, go ahead, and enjoy yourself. Try not to worry about myeloma."

Her countenance quickly changed. "Thank you so much," she said with a smile. "You've relieved my tension."

I was reluctant, however, to lose track of her again, and I emphasized the importance of regular follow-ups. "At the first sign of the M protein, we'll decide what to do," I said.

I still needed to tell her about one more recent option for myeloma in remission: using a new agent, Revlimid, as a maintenance drug. A maintenance drug keeps the cancer in check and prolongs remission, as with BMT. Approved in 2006 for myeloma treatment, it was a pioneering drug that modulates the patients' own immune system to kill the cancer cells.[2]

Since Revlimid was an oral medication, it was worth a try. Like other cancer

---

1 Despite its complexity and cost, BMT has been a lifesaver, at least for a while, for numerous select patients. With advances in transplant medicine, it has become safer than before. We owe much of the underlying idea, research, and practice about BMT to a Texas physician, E. Donall Thomas, the father of BMT, who was born in the tiny town of Mart in 1920. He received a Nobel Prize in Medicine in 1990. I met him once when he was at the height of his fame, and his humility humbled me.

2 The story of Revlimid, like the story of nitrogen mustard, is one more paradox in cancer medicine. It was derived from thalidomide, the hated drug that caused worldwide fear and horror in the 1950s and 1960s. Widely used as a sedative and morning sickness remedy, thalidomide induced severe birth defects in babies when taken by pregnant mothers. So, thalidomide was withdrawn from the market and banned in the US. Then, in the 1990s, it was found to be effective against myeloma. When oncologists prescribed it, the manufacturer required them to get a signed consent form from all women patients, regardless of age, to say that they weren't pregnant. Since most myeloma patients are above sixty, imagine their incredulity when they read the form. One eighty-two-year-old woman with MM gave me a strange look and blurted out, "You must be out of your mind, Doctor!"

drugs, it had drawbacks—the side effects. There was also another disabling, though nonmedical, toxicity to circumvent—its high cost: $8,000 per month. After her deductibles and out-of-pocket expenses, Clara's health insurance had covered her treatments before. But it balked at paying for Revlimid as a maintenance drug, since the FDA had yet to approve it as such. Later on, the price of Revlimid sharply increased to $22,000 per month when it was also approved for other diseases, such as myelodysplastic syndrome (a blood cancer) and certain lymphomas.

When she found out how much the medicine would cost and that she would have to pay the whole amount on her own, she asked me in frustration, "Do they think I'm Sam Walton, even if I'm willing to take it?"

Sam Walton, the billionaire co-founder of Walmart, had myeloma and died about two and a half years after his diagnosis. Understandably, his disease and death had been national news.

I searched for a solution for Clara. As things happen sometimes, she was one of those patients who fell through the cracks. She wasn't working, but her husband was. She had enough to live on but not enough to buy the dearly expensive medicines.

The pharmaceutical giants took notice of the outcry from doctors and patients about their exorbitant prices. The companies responded by saying that research and development are costly, as if they had performed these feats all by themselves. But that's far from the truth, as I explained in a forceful *New York Times* article on April 26, 1992, titled "The Public's Share of Medical Research."

Basic biomedical research has long been heavily subsidized by United States taxpayers. The federal government spends billions on the National Institutes of Health and gives numerous grants to universities to further research. High-tech pharmaceuticals owe their origin largely to these investments and to government scientists. The public has earned the right to buy the products at a reasonable price.

I reminded them in my article, "As a practicing physician, I wish I had better treatments for cancer patients. But what good is a superdrug if its cost is out of [our] reach?"

To pacify the public, Big Pharma came out with a patient-assistance program. But it applied to only a few of the suffering patients and required intrusive paperwork. The companies had more ways to deny than to accept. Even so, I asked Clara to give it a try.

"Let me talk to my family to see how I can go about it," she said.

While all this was going on, something else had begun to brew, and this was not about Clara but about me. It had been thirty-five years since I started my oncology practice, and I was thinking of retiring. When my colleagues heard about this, they had one reflexive thought—I was a casualty of physician burnout.

"I sympathize with you," a psychiatrist colleague said. "It's not easy to deal with a depressing specialty day in and day out. And dispensing poisons must be hard." Many others felt the same way.

By "poisons" they meant cancer drugs. What they were saying was common knowledge, especially in the early years of medical oncology, my specialty and the one responsible for chemotherapy. In contrast, surgical oncology fared better, and research oncology even had glamour. In some non-oncology circles, chemotherapy was even looked at with outright suspicion.

Three doctors in our town had left their practices in their late fifties because they were weighed down by burnout. Each echoed the same sentiment to me: "You see, Fazlur, I can't give my all to my patients when I feel this way."

My colleagues, however, were surprised by the truth of my own experience.

"I don't feel burnout," I said to them, "at least, not so far. I want to retire for personal reasons. The long hours don't leave me room for anything else. Retirement will give me more time with my family, and more time for my writing and teaching. Bureaucracy frustrates me, of course, as it does every doctor. And burnout is real and is a threat to our profession. But I've been lucky to escape it."

I must confess that I couldn't avoid a certain private struggle about my retirement decision. I wanted to go out in top form, which I believed myself to be in. In my professional life, I had seen doctors practice medicine beyond their time; they were out of date with medical advances, and I had to be extra careful when I saw their patients on consultation. On the other hand, some doctors, though still professionally sharp, practiced part-time in preparation for their retirement. Jack Rice, a urologist and close friend, six years older than I, had done so. "This made me feel useful as long as possible," he said, "and helped me to think about my coming years."

I understood what he meant by feeling "useful" when I broached my intent to retire with my patients. Many had been with me for years after their remission, and a few of them burst into tears and made me teary as well. I knew I would miss them all, and my daily life would be different without them. Moreover, in the process of my everyday work, I had to interact with so many colleagues, nurses, technicians, and ancillary personnel. It had been an engrossing career, and leaving it would be a drastic change.

Another friend, a respected former college president, advised me not to leave too soon. "You'll be miserable," he said. He had retired because of ill health, but he wasn't happy to leave the scene that made him what he was. Once he recovered, he went back into higher education.

While I was thinking over these different paths, I reached a point that seemed melodramatic even to myself when I started paraphrasing Hamlet: To retire, or not to retire, that is the question. Of course, I was far luckier than he—I wasn't a tortured soul, and I didn't have to take arms against a sea of troubles.

At a certain point, my past and present came together. Jahanara (Ara) and I grew up in what's now Bangladesh. I was from a village fifty miles east of Kolkata, India, and she was from a village near the remote Sundarbans. It was by a quirk of destiny that we met each other and fell in love. Then we had to part because of circumstances beyond our control.

We had faced our share of trials and tribulations from an early age, some of which I mentioned in the introduction. Ara struggled hard to get an education. Girls' schooling wasn't valued in the villages when she was a child. But she had her own mind and was determined to finish high school, and when she did, her father wanted to get her a husband. She again fought tradition and refused to wed any man she didn't love. Then, by sheer will and luck, we reconnected. We married in haste, risking our lives during a harsh curfew imposed by brutal Pakistani generals. Only a week after our wedding, I had no choice but to leave her once more to come to the United States. Later, fortune smiled upon us, and she was able to join me in New York after eighteen months, just before the outbreak of a vicious civil war in East Pakistan that led to the creation of Bangladesh in 1971.

During my long training and practicing years in New York, Houston, and San Angelo, Ara had to endure my frequent absence. Still, she left the retirement decision to me. She knew how much I loved my patients, and she felt uplifted whenever one of them saw her in the community and talked about me. We had little means when we started our lives together. It was my work that had given me not only professional rewards but also our financial security. Moreover, it had garnered us a name and a voice in society. I realized, however, that I couldn't ask for any more sacrifice from my life partner, and that clinched my decision to leave medicine.

With a heavy heart, I prepared my patients for my looming departure.

"I won't be seeing you any longer, Clara," I said to her during her last appointment. "I'll send you to my new colleague. He's a smart oncologist. He'll decide what to do about your maintenance treatment."

"So, you're letting him decide. That means he knows more than you," she said with a playful grin. Then she complimented me in her characteristic way: "I'll miss you if you go, but that's because I won't have a doctor to argue with. Don't change from what you are."

I wrote letters to all my patients: "I am deeply grateful to you for your trust in me, especially during your trying times, and for giving me the privilege of caring for you."

On my last day, I worked later than usual to say farewell to as many patients as I could. In the late evening, when everyone was gone and the place was quiet, I sat at my desk and closed my eyes, taking a moment to look back. I felt that trust and privilege more intensely than before. I didn't have adequate words to describe what I had witnessed in my patients all those years: Even while facing calamity, the human spirit has the gift for generosity. I consoled myself by accepting life as it is—when the time comes, one has to leave behind something one loves.

July 4 is a particularly special day for me. The birth of our nation and the birth of my daughter Gulshan fell on the same day. Moreover, it was on July 4, 2011, that the *San Angelo Standard-Times*, our daily paper, ran the front-page story on me and my retirement with the headline, "Doctor Retires with Love and Respect." The paper's reporter also wrote about my final hours in the hospital and office. She interviewed some of my patients and colleagues. In addition to others, she quoted one patient: "An older gentleman with a slow gait approached about closing time. He told the nurse he wanted to see Dr. Rahman, just to say goodbye. 'He did a lot for me the last few years. I will miss him. He is a kind, warm man.'"

How could I muster the means to express my gratitude for all the generosity I had received?

After I left, I began to write more of my memoir, parts of which had appeared before in the *Harvard Review* and the British medical journal with global reach, *The Lancet*, with other fragments here and there. The book was more consuming in time and thought than I had expected. It dredged up memories from my childhood—not only the painful ones, but also the happy times, and the enchanting myths and superstitions I grew up with. Working on the memoir helped me to understand better why I became a doctor and what made me the person I was, professionally and otherwise. My cultural and medical memoir, *The Temple Road: A Doctor's Journey*, was published in 2016 in Delhi, and it was well received and well reviewed throughout India and in a literary magazine in Singapore.

I also began to work in medical humanities and ethics, an area of my interest, as an advisory council member of the Charles E. Cheever Jr. Center for Medical Humanities and Ethics at the University of Texas Health Science Center in San Antonio. In addition, I taught the same subject in some semesters as an adjunct professor at Angelo State University. And I continued as a senior trustee of Austin College. All these endeavors made me feel useful outside my profession.

I didn't want to sever my old relations, however. On occasion, I visited my former oncologist colleague, Robert Prieto. He was well trained and caring, and before I left, I gladly transferred my patients, including Clara, to him.

He had stayed in San Angelo and established himself, which pleased me greatly. He had at first practiced with a big specialty group in San Antonio, but he sought a more intimate atmosphere and eventually contacted me. I was glad to invite him as my partner. Not many oncologists felt at home in remote West Texas; in the past, another hospital in town had gone through six oncologists, all of whom left for one reason or another. But Robert had been born and brought up in New Mexico at the West Texas border and was comfortable in San Angelo.

To my disappointment, I found out from Robert that Clara hadn't gone to him for follow-ups. I thought she likely hadn't survived, with such a high chance of fatal relapse.

Time seemed to pass without my notice. I went to see Robert again. He and I happened to meet each other in the hallway of his office. While exchanging pleasantries, I laughed out loud at something he said.

"I can recognize that laughter and accent anywhere," I heard a woman's voice say from a side room. "Come in here, please, Dr. Rahman." I went in, not sure who was there.

It was none other than Clara! Seeing my astonished stare, she said, "It's the real me, not my ghost."

Then, to needle me further, she said, "Have I fooled you again?"

She told me she had done neither the maintenance treatment nor the BMT. For that matter, she hadn't even seen an oncologist. Recently, she had had a bad respiratory infection, for which she was admitted to another hospital. After her discharge, she was referred to Dr. Prieto because of her myeloma history. She was still in remission.

"Why don't you write my story?" she said to me. "Others can learn from my illness. I'm a teacher, you know. I've liked your newspaper articles."

Over the years, I had written on medical, ethical, social, and personal issues for many national and international publications, including the *New York Times*, *Wall Street Journal*, *Guardian Weekly*, *Christian Science Monitor*, *Newsweek*, *Haaretz*, *Lancet*, and *Harvard Review*. Many of these articles were reprinted in regional papers, and Clara had read them in the *San Angelo Standard-Times*.

She jogged my memory.

"It was twenty-three years ago that you diagnosed my myeloma," she said, "and sent me to die in hospice."

She was still the same Clara, and she wasn't going to let me off without a witty remark. "Aren't you forgetting to harangue me about relapse?"

In later years, I thought of Clara off and on. She deepened my knowledge of human connection and partnership, with their complexities and tests. Moreover, how I dealt with my patients and how I interacted with them, especially in their most vulnerable moments, made a difference in their recovery and in my success and failure as their physician. These lessons were equally useful in navigating my daily life, grappling with my own adversities and those of my loved ones. Clara reinforced in my mind the value of hope and resilience in the face of bleakness.

Moreover, though I had only a limited encounter with Sandy Oliver in her short life—she was just thirty-six when she died of breast cancer—she, too, taught me something that's not taught in classes: grace under duress. Heaven knows how many times I failed her example.

Both patients have also compelled me to reflect on cancer's mysteries. Sure, we understand it better than we did when I first saw them, but we still have a long way to come out of the wilderness; we can't be too arrogant about our achievements. About ten million souls worldwide still die of cancer annually—every sixth death—and countless bear its brunt.

Why did these two women take two different paths? How do we explain that? We do have some textbook answers: one's tumor was sensitive to drugs and the other's wasn't. But again, why? We have a ready explanation for that, too—because of this mutation or that. But what prompted their normal cells to mutate to become malignant in the first place?

Clara is also a stark reminder to doctors that uncertainty, at times, works in our patients' favor, and a prognosis—good or bad—isn't written in stone.

PART 2

CORINA: WALKING A LONG PATH

CHAPTER 5

orina Johnson was admitted to the ICU through our ER because of shortness of breath. Though I was an oncologist, I was called in to see her. I was covering for the on-call internist who had to leave town suddenly due to a family crisis.

By the time I arrived at her bedside, her breathing had improved with oxygen. Despite her symptoms, she appeared calm and pleasant. A cancer doctor's presence without notice can be unnerving, so to avoid giving her unnecessary distress, I introduced myself as the on-call doctor rather than as an oncologist.

"How long have you had the breathing problem?" I asked.

"For the last two or three months, I've been getting slightly out of breath while working. I didn't pay much attention to it. I'm a cook in our school cafeteria, and I thought I was working too hard. I'm not young anymore—I turned sixty-two."

When her breathing didn't get any better, she went to her family doctor. "He said I had a respiratory infection with asthma and gave me medicines."

But Corina's symptoms progressed despite the medications. Her children were grown up and out of the home, and she hid her symptoms from her husband, a farmer, for as long as she could.

"It's plowing and sowing time," she said. "He starts his work before daylight and doesn't stop until dark. He comes home dead tired and goes to sleep early. Farming is difficult these days for small farmers—too much work and too little money. Without my school job, we wouldn't make it."

I opened her gown to examine her chest. She bore the scars of a radical mastectomy—a prominent scar where her right breast had been—and her right arm had lymphedema, swelling caused by blockage of the lymphatic circulation. I found out that she had that surgery in the 1950s, when radical mastectomy, regardless of the size of the breast tumor, was the standard operation. It was a drastic and disfiguring procedure: removal of the whole breast along with the chest muscles and dozens of axillary lymph nodes. And lymphedema was a common, mostly incurable aftereffect. In some patients, the swelling was massive and disabling, curtailing their quality of life, even when their cancer was gone.

Corina's chest x-ray showed pleural effusion in the right lung, but the left lung was clear. The pleura is a protective, two-layer membrane around each lung. Pleural effusion is the collection of fluid between these layers. Several conditions can produce the fluid, but with her history, it indicated an alarming cause: pleural metastasis from breast cancer. I had to temper my thinking, however; it had been twenty-six years since her cancer diagnosis.

"Did you tell the ER doctor about your mastectomy?" I asked her.

"No one asked me about my surgery. It was so long ago that I've forgotten it myself. I was only thirty-six then. My surgeon told me he'd taken out all the cancer and not to worry about it anymore. So, I've kept it out of my mind."

Pleural fluid presses on the affected lung, leading to shortness of breath. Thus, the first thing to do was to drain the fluid so that Corina's lung could expand and she could breathe more easily. Then, I would send the fluid to the lab for analysis.

I inserted a tube into her fluid cavity and removed as much fluid as I could. Then, the tube was connected to a plastic bag to drain the remaining effusion. She was surprised how quickly her breathing eased.

Because her effusion had built up slowly, she had been able to handle it and continue her job, until she reached a threshold when her lung became so squeezed that she had asthma-like respiration. That's what had brought her to the hospital.

Two days later, Martin Kulig, a pathologist colleague, gave me a report on the fluid. "It has malignant cells compatible with breast cancer." Sometimes cancer cells aren't easy to detect in an effusion, but Martin was a keen-eyed observer, and I could rely on his judgment.

So far, I had kept quiet about my concern. I wished I were Corina's internist, because then I could have referred her to an oncologist. She still thought asthma and respiratory infection had brought on the effusion and the symptoms. She asked me to send her home since she was breathing well.

"I'm sorry," I said. "You aren't ready to be discharged."

"Why? You've taken out the fluid."

"Your relief is temporary. I'm afraid it'll come back soon unless we treat the real problem."

"What problem?"

I gently said, "I'm sorry, your breast cancer has spread to the covering of your lung. It's the cancer that has produced the fluid, and it'll keep making it until the cancer is controlled."

Her eyes went wide with disbelief. "How can that be? My surgeon cut out all the cancer. He reassured my husband and me that I was cured."

"I know what you mean." Then I explained that I was a cancer doctor and, by coincidence, had been on call when she came into the ER.

She was so dumbfounded that she didn't pay attention to the doctor part.

"It doesn't make sense," she murmured.

Her doubt was understandable. At the time of her surgery, the behavior of breast cancer was poorly understood. Surgeons erroneously believed that radical mastectomy, a brutal operation, was the way to cure it. And they routinely told their patients as much, or at least their patients were left with that impression. Besides, there was social chauvinism at play. Doctors at that time often assumed that women weren't equipped to handle a cancer diagnosis. Therefore, they informed only the patients' husbands or male relatives. Rachel Carson, the author of *Silent Spring*, was a famous example of this travesty. After she had a radical mastectomy in 1960 for breast cancer, her surgeon lied to her about the diagnosis when she asked.

"Did my surgeon make some mistake?" Mrs. Johnson asked after she recovered.

"Of course not. He did take out the cancer with the mastectomy."

"Why is it back, then?"

I gave her a simple explanation about breast cancer relapse. A few of the cancer cells escape from the tumor and stay dormant inside the body. Surgeons can remove only what they can see, and you can't see cancer cells with the naked eye. In time, the dormant cells become active and can settle anywhere and grow.

"In your case, the cancer has come back in the covering of the right lung," I said. "We need to perform more tests and then decide what to do."

It so happened that I had come to know Corina's surgeon during the waning years of his practice. He was an accomplished doctor and had referred a dozen or so breast cancer patients to me. I decided to call him with an update on Corina's status, even though I wasn't sure if he would remember her—he had seen her only a few times since the operation twenty-six years before.

"I haven't forgotten her," he said. "How could I? She was a young woman with children. You don't see too many breast cancers at her age."

"She's here with pleural metastasis with effusion. She's understandably shocked that her cancer is back after so many years. She thought she was cured by the surgery."

I shouldn't have said that last sentence.

"What was I expected to tell her?" he said defensively. "That she had incurable cancer? That would make her miserable as long as she lived. She was so young and was raising kids. At least in terms of her cancer, she was at peace all these years."

I couldn't argue with him on that point, especially since there wasn't much to offer at the time besides surgery and radiation. But radiation, like surgery, had its limits; you controlled only the local disease on the chest wall. Besides, unlike some doctors, he had mentioned the diagnosis to the patient herself.

I had no control over what had happened in the past. Corina and I were bound to the present, and it was the present that we had to deal with. Breast cancer commonly spreads to the bones, lungs, and liver. Doctors had a small number of tests available to guide them when Corina was first diagnosed, such as ordinary bone and liver scans and plain x-rays (no CT or MRI yet).

To our relief, Corina's other tests were normal. Her metastasis, therefore, was confined to the pleura only, and the lungs themselves were free of tumors. I explained everything I had found and talked about treatment with two available choices: hormones and chemotherapy.

"Hormone treatment sounds familiar," she said. "Which hormone?"

"Estrogen."

"Estrogen!" she said in surprise. "My doctor me told not to take it. Isn't it bad for breast cancer?"

Both she and I were right. The reason she was advised to avoid estrogen was because at the standard low dose, it stimulates breast cancer cells, while at a high dose, it kills them. This is known as—what else—the "estrogen paradox." I went through all this with her.

"I'll take the hormone then," she said.

She had also heard about chemotherapy, which, in her mind, was dangerous. I hated to disappoint her again, but I had to explain that high-dose estrogen (HDE) isn't benign. It's fraught with adverse effects, such as congestive heart failure, nausea and vomiting, vaginal bleeding, and thromboembolism. I had witnessed most of these side effects in my patients. Some patients felt so wretched on HDE that they gave up the hormone and took their chances with the cancer. But until the FDA approved the groundbreaking hormone Tamoxifen in 1978, HDE was a common drug for metastatic breast cancer.

"That doesn't sound good," she said. "You seem against it."

"I prefer a new chemotherapy called CMF," I said. "It's a combination of three drugs with long names: cyclophosphamide, methotrexate, and 5-fluorouracil, or 5-FU."

To avoid overburdening her with all the information at once, I added, "You don't need to remember the names. I'll give you simple booklets to read. After reading them, you can ask me any questions. I also need one of your family members to hear about the treatment plan. That way the person can remind you if you forget something."

"I can get my daughter-in-law, Cindy," Corina said. "My son is working in an oil field far away, in Iraan in Pecos County. Harold, my husband, can't handle this sort of thing. He's a nervous man. He went to pieces when my cancer was first diagnosed, and we were young then. All he does is farming, and I take care of the rest. This may sound odd to you, but he's lost without me. I need to be around a little longer. Cindy takes things well and she's good to me."

I hadn't met her husband yet. The nurses had told me that he had come and gone but hadn't asked for me. I knew that family members tended to have diverse temperaments. Some got intimately involved with their loved ones' care, while others, though dutiful, stayed aloof to cope in their own way.

Cindy came to the hospital to help her mother-in-law, and she, too, had the usual fear of chemo. Both women understood the gravity of what was at hand, and they asked me questions. They were mainly worried about how the treatment would affect Corina.

"Different patients react to chemo differently," I said. "Those who're physically active tend to tolerate chemo better than those who are sedentary. You've been doing physical work for so many years, you should handle it well." I elaborated on how chemo works and its benefits and side effects.

"Why three drugs at a time?" Cindy asked.

"The cells in our body have various stages of growth until they mature. Cells in a tumor are also the same way. Different drugs work at different stages, so if we combine them, we can kill all the cells in a tumor."

The CMF regimen could be administered in various ways. Simply going by the book doesn't always work in chemo because it's a long-haul treatment, routinely given for months, and sometimes for years. Therefore, at times, you have to accommodate the patient so that they can comply with what's possible for them. The best chemo is of no use if patients are unable to take it for practical reasons.

West Texas is a far-flung area, and cancer patients were often referred to me from as far away as the far end of Big Bend, 300 miles southwest of San Angelo. Corina lived in a distant part of the countryside, and she would have to drive three hours each way to come see me. Plus, she wanted to keep working in between her chemos. The treatment also had a complicated schedule, with oral tablets and IV injections at regular intervals; the whole cycle was then repeated every month as long as the chemo was effective. But psychologically, it wasn't easy to wake up every morning to take chemo tablets and experience nausea, especially if you had to function at your job.

The CMF regimen, however, had changed with time, and the schedule for Corina would be all three drugs administered intravenously in one sitting, with the cycle repeated every three weeks. Not only was this schedule more convenient, but it was also more tolerable. Patients received IV medications during the chemo to prevent nausea and vomiting. After the chemo was done at the clinic, they were sent home with antinausea tablets.

Corina started the three-weekly regimen. Although her nausea was under control, she couldn't avoid the other side effects, including myelosuppression—bone marrow suppression—resulting in low blood counts. I titrated the chemo doses to find an optimum level that tempered the degree of myelosuppression. In reality, chemotherapy is not only a trial for patients but also a juggling act for oncologists. Since the idiosyncratic biology of a tumor and its individual sufferer warrant specific attention, the treatment of some metastatic cancers is no place to rigidly follow a set of stringent rules.

I hadn't forgotten my lessons learned from the zealotry that characterized the early years of clinical oncology. In the name of preventing infections from outside sources, we put our patients through some miserable measures. We routinely placed them in strict isolation in the hospital rooms, severely restricted visitors, and allowed only certain nurses to attend to them. This demoralized the patients and put strain on the nurses, who had to deal with burdensome rules. Worse, patients were given prophylactic oral antibiotics to eradicate the bacteria in their gut, in the hope of averting infections from these organisms.

Because many of the infections in these patients come not from outside but from the microbes that are normally present in our body, it turned out that the measures did more harm than good. As stated before, these germs are harmless to healthy persons, but they attack hosts whose blood counts and immunity are dangerously low. To complicate the matter further, the oral antibiotics eliminated the good bacteria, giving the bad ones the upper hand. Hence, the strict methods were a futile exercise. In retrospect, standard hygienic practices—good handwashing and use of sterile gloves, masks, and gowns—would have been sufficient.

In the course of her chemo, Corina told me about part of her life. She presented it like a storyteller. Sometimes she expressed herself that way later on as well. Though this took time out of my day, I enjoyed her style.

"My husband and I grew up in the Depression. We scraped to put food on the table. But we were farmers and were luckier than most since we could grow things. Many people we knew almost starved. We helped each other as much as we could, but there wasn't much to share. Shops and stores were closed, and clerks and secretaries were laid off. Some people felt so humiliated that they suffered terribly rather than ask for charity."

My former friends and colleagues in Houston cautioned me before moving to San Angelo: "If you live out in the country, you'll have to put up with boring farmers and farmwives." Nothing could have been further from the truth.

Eventually, Corina shared how her breast cancer had been initially diagnosed.

"It couldn't have happened at a worse time or in a worse way," she said. "We had three little kids and were struggling to make a living. Farming wasn't going well—the cotton crop was poor that year. And it was one of those times of bad drought that regularly hits West Texas. In the middle of all this, I felt a lump in my right breast. My family doctor sent me to a surgeon. He took out the lump under general anesthesia. When I woke up, he gave me good news: I didn't have cancer. I thanked God and went home with gratitude. My husband and I were so happy."

She paused a moment, and then, with moist eyes, continued. "Two days later, the surgeon called me. I thought it was nice of him to check on me. Instead, he said, 'I'm sorry, the final pathology report is different—you have cancer in the breast. You must have surgery now to save your life.' Next week he did what he called a radical mastectomy and told us I was cured."

She was right about the ways of breast cancer diagnosis and surgery in the 1950s through the 1970s. A breast lump was biopsied under general anesthesia. After that, the pathologist did a quick study of the specimen to look for cancer, while the patient was still under anesthesia on the operating table and the surgeon was waiting. If no cancer was found, surgery was avoided, and the patient was sent home. Regardless of the results of the quick study, all the specimens were also verified with what's called a "permanent section," the most accurate method of cancer diagnosis; this required two to three days. If the cancer was missed with the quick method, it was found in the permanent section. The patient was then called back for surgery.

All this took place because the quick method had shortcomings: on occasion, it gave false-negative and false-positive results. The false-negative patients, like Corina, had to undergo general anesthesia again to have the radical mastectomy. And the other unfortunate ones were the false positives. The mastectomies were done right then and there if the quick method found cancer, but then, later, the permanent section showed no cancer at all. The women had undergone an unnecessary surgery and had lost a breast for no good reason. In my early years, I saw all this firsthand. When the patients went to surgery, they had no way of knowing ahead of time if they would wake up from anesthesia with or without a breast. This uncertainty was nerve-wracking.

What a world of change has taken place in the breast cancer field since then. Patients now undergo a needle biopsy with local anesthesia right in the x-ray department if a mammogram shows a suspicious lump. This tiny specimen is sent to the lab for detailed studies, which include looking for the tumor's estrogen, progesterone, and HER 2 receptors and genetic footprints. The results tell us whether the cancer is a good or a poor prognostic type. Patients know all this ahead of the operation and are given treatment choices, including the type of surgery, knowing that removing the breast alone may not be sufficient. About 80 percent of the patients have only a lumpectomy—resection of the cancerous segment only—preserving the breast, and the rest have a modified radical mastectomy, which is less disfiguring than the old radical mastectomy and has no subsequent lymphedema. This is a far cry from not knowing whether the patients would wake up from anesthesia with or without a breast. And, it prevents the heartbreak from the false results.

CHAPTER 6

orina's side effects from the chemo were fewer than usual. "All your physical activity is helping you now," I said to her.

"I've done plenty of that," she said. "It's not just working in the kitchen at my job. I've worked in the fields side by side with my husband, in good weather and bad. On weekends, when school is out, I dig postholes and build fences on the farm. Quite a few women in farming country do these kinds of things." I knew that digging postholes and building fences were strenuous labor, especially in the blazing West Texas summer.

The lymphedema in Corina's right arm wasn't as bad as I had seen in others. Her surgeon had skill, and also, her high activity level may have helped her lymphatic circulation. She was a woman of small stature with a gentle face and mild manner, and her hair was arranged in a neat bun. And she was a down-to-earth person. Her external features might mislead you about how strong she was.

She followed my instructions well. She ate at least some food, even when her appetite was low. Cyclophosphamide (CP) can induce cystitis, causing pain and urinary bleeding. This happens when CP sits in the bladder after being cleared by the kidneys. To prevent this, patients must drink plenty of liquid and empty their bladder often. Corina did both.

She responded to chemo well, and after the third cycle, her residual effusion resolved. As she got her energy back, she went back to her job in between treatments.

"I don't like to miss work," she said. "It puts an extra burden on my friends in the kitchen. Several of the girls have young children."

There was something else she longed for: "I've gotten used to the hustle and bustle of the school kids. I miss them."

How long should we continue chemo for metastatic cancer like hers? Give it as long as it works, or stop once we achieve complete remission? Things weren't clear cut yet.

"Your fluid is gone," I said to her. "We have to decide what to do next. Let me refer you to MD Anderson Cancer Center for a second opinion."

"We're country folks," she said. "We aren't comfortable going to Houston—too big and too far away. You do what you can here."

This was a common sentiment among those who lived in the country. San Angelo, then with 70,000 people, was big enough for them. Besides, Houston was 400 miles away. As a compromise, I called a friend at MD Anderson to discuss her issue—Gabriel Hortobagyi, a rising star in the breast cancer department.

"So far, her options are limited," Gabriel said, "unless she wants to take part in clinical trials." Corina and I had already talked about a trial, and she had declined it for practical reasons.

I ended up keeping Corina on chemo for a year and a half. Chemo side effects being cumulative—the more chemo you take, the more side effects you get—we watched her closely. Besides, CP is also a leukemogenic agent, a drug that can mutate the cells in the marrow and incite leukemia. Of course, that's not the primary concern for patients whose lifespan is limited, as with most metastatic cancers, for it takes time for the mutation to take place. But it's a worry for those who are curable or expected to survive for years.

Side effects aside, the realities of daily life come into play during chemo. Visiting the oncologist every three weeks, getting stuck with needles for chemo, and then experiencing nausea and more are no walk in the park. Especially since we didn't have as good antinausea medications, oral or IV, then. Corina's recurrent hardships were shared by most patients: get chemo and become transiently sick, feel well once the acute side effects are gone, then return for the next round of chemo and repeat the cycle of sickness all over again.

There were also other burdens to bear. Doctors order regular blood counts for patients on chemo, as well as periodic x-rays and scans to check the response to treatment. Obviously, if the cancer is advancing despite the treatment, the treatment has to be stopped. Besides, on occasion, some patients end up in the hospital for one complication or another.

Frustrations can also build up in other ways. Concomitant non-chemo drugs have side effects, too. Patients may get drowsy from the antiemetics given with the chemo, so they require someone to drive them back and forth to the doctors and labs. This dependence on others, including family members and friends, can be disruptive, especially if the helpers hold jobs. It's easy for others to be generous once in a while or for a limited time, but it's hard to be charitable month after month.

I had my own worry along the way: the possibility of stealthy chemo resistance, before it even showed up as tumor progression. This is more the case for tumors that are less responsive; for example, Hodgkin's disease is more sensitive to chemo than breast cancer. Yet, breast cancer is more responsive than, say, colon cancer.

Could I give Corina some kind of maintenance treatment to keep her in remission? If the maintenance chemo was harmful, what about a non-chemo agent? My reservations about the high-dose estrogen (HDE) aside, it hadn't been used as a maintenance drug. Oncologists also utilized another hormone, testosterone—the male counterpart of estrogen—to treat metastatic breast cancer. Since breast tumor is estrogen-dependent, countering the effects of the estrogen would suppress the tumor, and testosterone would surely do that. But, as with HDE, there is a price to pay. Testosterone has virilizing effects, including acne and a change in the voice, which acquires a male tone. More troublesome is hirsutism—unwanted male-pattern hair growth in women, with excessive coarse hair on the face, chest, and back.

I wasn't totally opposed to HDE or testosterone. They had their places. But I found that only select patients agreed to continue either of these hormones for long. It was best to leave Corina alone without a maintenance treatment.

To save Corina hours of driving, I asked her to follow up with her local physician. I saw her again after four months. She looked like a new person. Her alopecia from chemo was gone, and her hair had grown back. "I have a new hairstyle," she said. "It's short and naturally curly." She had the so-called "chemo curl." Its exact mechanism is ill understood. Cyclophosphamide and similar drugs injure the hair follicles, which is why the hair falls out during chemo. Once the chemo effects end, the altered follicles produce curls in the process of regrowing the hair.

Since Corina had been a captive of chemo for eighteen months, I was happy that her life was back to normal.

About three months later, I got a call from an orthopedist colleague, Price Burdine, in the middle of the night. "I have Corina Johnson here in the hospital," he said. Then I heard an urgent voice in the background. "Hold on a minute, Fazlur," he said. "I need to find out what's going on."

I knew that being called at that hour by a colleague, especially an orthopedic surgeon, wasn't a good sign. I dreaded any news of pathologic fractures from metastatic cancer. Since bone fragility because of the cancer was a factor, some of these fractures were difficult to fix. Not only that—after the surgery, patients still needed radiation on the operated site to get rid of the residual cancer.

While waiting for the orthopedist to return to the phone, thoughts flashed through my mind: had Corina's cancer come back? It would be so unfair if it did. Just a few months ago, she looked content and well. And if she had a fracture, was it in one or more places? With multiple fractures, her days could be numbered.

Besides the possible surgical problems, the likely post-op complications worried me. I had seen enough of them—in particular, thromboembolism and infection. And if they both happen simultaneously, you have to juggle the treatments. You manage the clots with blood-thinning medicine, and you fret about bleeding in the vital organs. Then you give strong antibiotics to control infection—ordinary antibiotics are often ineffective in immunosuppressed patients—and you become anxious about damaging the kidneys.

As minutes ticked by on the phone, I forced myself to find something positive. Price Burdine had good hands and good judgment, the hallmark of a superior surgeon. His operative complications were low, and he had been practicing for years. My patients had fared well with his surgery.

Burdine picked up the phone again. "Sorry, Fazlur, for keeping you waiting. Corina has a fracture of the neck of the left femur, with contusions here and there. I can't tell from her history which came first—the fall and then the fracture, or the other way around."

He was making a crucial point about clinical suspicion. The injury he was describing was a hip fracture—the weakest part of the hip is the neck of the femur. If Corina's fracture had occurred because of a fall, the bone broke from the impact of the trauma; in that case, she had a traumatic fracture, a common occurrence among the elderly. But if a spontaneous breakage caused her to fall, she likely had a pathological fracture. The problem is that patients can't always tell what happened when.

"I've seen her x-rays," Burdine added. "The bones look mostly healthy, but with her cancer history, I have to make sure. I'll get a femoral tomogram in the morning."

A tomogram involves x-raying an object section by section to get a close-up view of any abnormality. These were the plain x-ray tomograms of the old days, before the arrival of CT and MRI. Now, tomography with CT and MRI is used not only in everyday medical practice but also for imaging in other sciences, such as archaeology, biology, geophysics, astrophysics, and materials science.

There was a ray of hope in Burdine's comment that the bones looked mostly healthy. At least he didn't outright call it a pathological fracture. This eased my anxiety.

"Do you want me to come to see her now?" I asked him.

"There's nothing for you to do tonight. You can see her in the morning when you make your rounds. I'm calling to give you a heads-up."

He knew that I was the only oncologist for the town and the whole region, and I was taking calls almost every night. Less-confident surgeons would have behaved differently. A few of them would have asked me to see the patient right then; they were unsure of taking care of patients with a history of chemo, regardless of the simplicity or complexity of the current condition. Others would have said, "It's up to you whether you want to come now or later." The latter would give me concern and make me lie in bed fitfully, and I would then disturb my sleeping wife and leave for the hospital. Reassurance from a colleague you respect has great value.

Five hours later, in the early morning, I was with Corina.

"I didn't think it'd come to this after fighting my cancer," she said. "I never had such excruciating pain in my life. The breast operation did give me a lot of pain, but not like this."

Analgesics had reduced her pain, and she was alert enough to tell me her story in her usual style.

"It rained last evening after a whole year, and I was happy that our cotton crop wouldn't die. I went to the barn to make sure our cows were all right. When I got back from the barn and was going into my house, I must've gotten careless. I slipped on the wet stairs and was half inside and half outside the door. I knew I'd broken something when the pain hit me hard and I couldn't move. I screamed again and again, but no one heard me. I lay there helpless."

She stopped to control her emotions, then began again. "My husband was out of town on farm business. My neighbors live a bit away. Harold was supposed to call and let me know how things were going. He phoned me at night. I could hear the ringing but there was nothing I could do. When he wasn't able to reach me, he called a friend. The friend found me and dialed 911. An ambulance took me to the emergency room. I stayed there for quite a while for x-rays and labs. By the time Dr. Burdine checked me, it was about midnight."

Then, she added, "I wouldn't live anywhere except the country, but it's not as easy as it looks."

I wanted to make sure there was no cancer in the fractured bone, so I talked to the pathologist ahead of the operation and gave Corina's history. Since pathologists don't know the patients firsthand—the only ones they have direct contact with are cadavers that need autopsy—they appreciate the clinician's information for making a diagnosis, especially in difficult cases. (One pathologist colleague used to joke, "I went into pathology so that I don't have to spend my days hearing complaints. Do you think cadavers complain?")

Dr. Burdine replaced Corina's fractured hip. The surgery went well, and the pathologist confirmed the clinical findings—no malignancy. Perhaps my undue apprehension was misplaced.

Corina's stoicism and attitude didn't fail her. She recovered uneventfully from her operation, and she accepted the rigors of rehab without quibble. Her only objection was what was true to her spirit: "I'm not useful to my family or to my coworkers."

In about ten weeks, she was back to her active life, with some limitations. "I can't do much heavy work anymore," she said. "Harold won't even let me try. And my daughter-in-law keeps tabs on me. She and my son moved away because of his work in the oil fields. After my accident, they've moved back near our farm."

During one follow-up, she talked more about a friend than about herself. "She had cancer of the ovary," Corina said. "She had a long operation and was deathly ill from a blocked bowel. They kept her in the hospital in Lubbock for weeks. When she came home, she was still very weak and quite down. I spent a few days with her to help her to pick up the pieces."

That was Corina Johnson's way. This wasn't the first time she had brought up the medical problems of her neighbors and friends. I admired her concern for others and the way she gave them a helping hand. It was one thing to hear her own story, but quite another to hear the stories of people with whom I had no connection. If I happened to be pressed for time, these external conversations frustrated me—more so when she asked for my opinion about their treatments. But I did my best to hide this feeling from her.

On another visit, she told me about one more friend. "He had lung cancer and went downhill fast and didn't make it. He was a good man and a good farmer. I wonder if the doctors did the right thing. I wish he came to you."

What she was opining isn't uncommon. If patients like a doctor, they want their friends and relatives to see that physician. What's forgotten is that sometimes it is the nature of the disease—not the doctor's lack of competence—that determines the fate of the patient. Although I was grateful for her faith in me, I had to tell her about the limits of my medical prowess.

"You and your friend had two completely different problems."

"Of course, I know, breast cancer and lung cancer."

"There's more to it than that. Lung cancer is one of the most difficult cancers to treat. There's not much one can do for a lung cancer that has spread."

"Thanks for telling me. My friend didn't say much. He kept to himself and smoked a lot."

"Some people are reluctant to talk to others about their cancer. Even to friends."

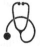

A few months later, I got a call from Corina's supervisor at work. "Corina doesn't look good," she said. "She has pain in her abdomen and still has come to work. I know about your giving her permission to work. But if you can tell me about her prognosis, I can help her out."

"I'm sorry," I said. "I can't divulge medical information without her consent."

"I'm aware of that, Dr. Rahman, but my problem is that she's more concerned about her coworkers than about herself. I wish I could say that about a few of the others in my department."

Then I remembered that Corina had told me I could talk to her supervisor if she inquired. But I had forgotten to ask my nurse to get a consent form signed. I felt caught in the middle. Living in big cities for so many years, I was trying to get used to certain West Texas ways. With some West Texans, word and honor are connected, and one's word was enough to be honored without a paper. While I was silent and thinking, the supervisor sensed my hesitation and added, "I understand your concern for privacy, but Corina asked me to call you. I know she needs to keep her job."

It was a time when it was easy to find excuses to get rid of employees with illnesses. I once took care of a woman in her early forties who was a valued legal assistant for a law firm out of town that specialized in malpractice lawsuits. She had sarcoma of a muscle and was on chemo after her surgery. She still worked between her treatments. One day, she came to me in tears.

"I've given twenty years of my life to them," she said. "I became a top assistant and a trusted hand. I took a lot of courses to keep up to date. I knew the cases inside out, sometimes more than some of our lawyers did. I suggested which cases should be settled and which should go to trial. Now they treat me like dirt. They fired me because I missed work on the chemo days." She had no recourse to fight back.

Yet, Corina's supervisor was bending over backward to keep her employee. Even with her health insurance, Corina had plenty of costs and deductibles. Also, cancer care isn't a one-shot deal; after the treatment is completed, there are years of follow-ups with doctors, as well as labs, x-rays, and scans. And that doesn't even include costly medicines for cancer and other concomitant diseases, such as diabetes, hypertension, and arthritis. Taken together, out-of-pocket expenses add up to a great deal.

"I appreciate your kindness to Corina," I told the supervisor. "Please ask her to see me. I need to check her abdomen. After that, I can tell you what you want to know."

CHAPTER 7

orina Johnson didn't like to complain, so when she did, I was more fearful than usual. And her supervisor was right about her ways—she came to work despite her abdominal pain. On examination, I felt a mass in the left upper quadrant of the abdomen. What could it be? A primary colon cancer? More worrisome—breast cancer can also metastasize to the colon as it can to anywhere else.

The means for diagnosing cancer had improved throughout the years, and by that time, CT scans were available. I ordered an abdominal CT and asked a radiologist colleague to give me a verbal report as soon as possible.

"There's a mass in the colon at the splenic flexure," he said. "But I'm not sure if it's cancer." I walked to the radiology department and looked at the scan with him. It was a peculiar mass inside the colon, above the spleen. It's not commonly known that with every new medical technology, there is a learning curve for doctors, and it takes practice to become skilled at it; it doesn't matter whether it's the latest scan or robotic surgery. When it comes to this issue, experts at the big cancer centers are no different from other doctors. The CT scan, being a recent development at that time, was at that stage.

"The best way to settle this is to have a colonoscopy," I told Corina. She agreed, with a positive note: "At least you haven't said it's surely a cancer."

The preparation for a colonoscopy—cleansing the bowel—was more taxing than the procedure itself. You had to drink tons of fluids and take a large amount of laxatives, and for the twenty-four hours preceding the colonoscopy, you were forced to frequent the bathroom day and night. If the colon wasn't clear, the colonoscopist couldn't visualize any lesions, and they could miss the diagnosis. For weak patients, the whole process was difficult. Corina did her best to follow the protocol.

The gastroenterologist talked to me as soon as he finished.

"I didn't see anything wrong," he said. "There's no colonic lesion to biopsy."

"No lesion?" I asked. "There's an obvious palpable mass, and you saw it on the CT."

He sensed the doubt in my voice.

"That's the trouble with you oncologists," he shot back. "Every headache must be a brain tumor."

"What do you think the mass is, then?"

"There's a simple explanation. She had bad constipation and had a hard stool ball in the splenic flexure that obstructed her colon. That's the reason for her abdominal pain. It was the stool ball, not a tumor, that we felt and saw. All the laxatives she took for the colon-prep softened it, and she passed it out as liquid stool. I've seen several cases like this before."

His explanation made sense and reminded me of an incident in the 1970s, when I was a senior medical resident at Baylor College of Medicine in Houston. A second-year medical student was under my supervision. The CT scan was still an "experimental" procedure, and my student took part in the control group as a healthy subject. It wasn't uncommon for us to volunteer as healthy controls or to give blood for lab experiments. Sometimes we even got paid for these services; with our low stipends, we were always short of money.

One day, my student showed up with an ashen, frightened face. I asked him what was bothering him.

"I'm doomed for good, Dr. Rahman," he said. "How am I going to explain this to my parents?" He was fighting not to cry.

He'd had an abdominal CT that morning as a control and was found to have a lump near the head of the pancreas along the colon, consistent with pancreatic cancer. Delving into his textbook, he found that his diagnosis essentially meant a death sentence. I couldn't believe what was in store for him and felt deeply sad. "It must be a mistake," I consoled him. He was to have a repeat CT scan the next day. I hoped and prayed that the reading of the first CT was wrong.

He panicked after his diagnosis and had diarrhea the whole time. When he came to the ward in the late morning, his eyes were sunken and discolored from dehydration and exhaustion. Strangely though, he was all smiles. Medical students sometimes have odd reactions to signs and symptoms. Had the fatal diagnosis deranged his mind? Or something else on top of that? Fortunately, it was nothing of the kind. The pancreatic mass, again, was apparently a compacted fecal ball and was flushed out by the diarrhea. His colon was clear after that, and his second CT was normal. I asked him to take the day off and drink plenty of fluids.

My gastroenterologist colleague had reason to take my initial doubt personally. Like all doctors, some colonoscopists are more adroit than others. I had known one who bragged that he was the "fastest in the West." Every day, he went from one procedure to another in rapid succession until he reached his quota, though this entailed the risk of missing something subtle. Hospitals liked him because he brought in plenty of revenue.

But Corina's gastroenterologist adhered to a sound colonoscopic principle: the more time you take to inspect the colonic lumen, the lower your chance of missing a lesion.

I reflected on Corina's two setbacks—the fracture and the abdominal mass—and how they'd turned out. How many times could she get lucky?

"Do you always worry like this?" she asked me. "Can't cancer patients have other things?"

I didn't have a good answer to her first question, but the second one was easy. "Yes, you're right, cancer patients can get other illnesses like everyone else."

"I've stopped worrying too much about myself," she said. "I've got a loving husband. My son and daughter are adults with families, and they're independent. And my five grandchildren are healthy and happy. Even with my cancer, I feel blessed."

I admired her outlook on living, and I could understand what made her calm despite her tribulations. Something more emerged from her when it came to her husband, something selfless: she wanted to survive not so much for herself as for him.

"He gets lost outside farming," she said to me again. "I don't know what'll happen to him without me. I'm the one who takes care of money, writes all the checks, and pays the bills. I've also learned to ask for bank loans to buy seeds, but since banks won't talk to a woman about loans without her husband there, he has to come with me."

Corina's comment about my worrying too much had an effect on my approach to patients. It reminded me of the admonition of Professor S. M.

Rab, my mentor in medical school: "Patients pick up from your demeanor how you feel about them and their illnesses. Remember, healing begins with your empathy and your reassuring presence at the bedside."

The results of many new breast cancer studies were steadily being published. One important discovery concerned the estrogen and progesterone receptors in breast cancer cells. If they are positive—that is, if the receptors are present in the malignant cells—anti-estrogens are effective in both prevention and treatment. Naturally, we needed good anti-estrogens, better than the unloved testosterone and high-dose estrogen. One unique drug of the anti-estrogen class is Tamoxifen, which was widely publicized when it arrived on the market. In the cancer field, investigators' initial zeal in touting a "breakthrough" doesn't often pan out. But not in the case of Tamoxifen, or Tam. It was, in my mind, a godsend, the kind of anti-estrogen I was looking for. The FDA approved it in 1978, and it has saved, and continues to save, countless lives. It works for prevention, treatment, and maintenance.

Tam is one of the cheapest medicines, cancer drug or not. It costs as little as sixty cents for a day's dose. That's why its impact is immense, because according to the World Health Organization (WHO), breast cancer is the most common malignancy around the globe. In 2020, 2.3 million cases were diagnosed worldwide, and 7.8 million women lived with a breast cancer diagnosis. For poor women everywhere, in developing countries in particular, Tam is a blessing. It's on the WHO's list of essential cancer medicines for all countries. We owe this boon to another Texas-born scientist, V. Craig Jordan, the father of Tam, born in New Braunfels in 1947.

No drug comes without side effects and neither did Tam. But almost all patients tolerated it well. It helped that it was a tablet, not an injection, and it was easy to take—just one or two tablets daily.

Since one recurrence of cancer is a harbinger of another, I was happy to have something to give Corina to forestall relapse. She accepted the new drug, even though she had no evidence of cancer at the time. Except for minor hot flashes and some weight gain, she had no other problems. She agreed to continue Tam for an indefinite period. How long to continue it in cases like hers hadn't yet been worked out. After two years, we settled into a routine—I would see her every six months. We were both gratified by her good luck. When she reached a significant milestone—five years of remission—she was able to be seen by her family practitioner (FP) only.

One night, about a year later, a frantic telephone call woke me up.

"Corina is very sick, Dr. Rahman," a man's voice said. "She can't breathe. She's sweating and her heart is pounding. I'm afraid the fluid in her lung has come back."

It was her husband who was on the line. In those years before cell phones, my chemotherapy patients had my home number to call in case of nighttime emergencies.

I tried to reassure Harold. "Maybe it's asthma," I said. Corina did have some form of ill-defined mild asthma. It showed up during the high pollen season of cedars, which are bountiful in West Texas.

Harold disagreed with me. "Her asthma never acted like this."

"Please get her to the hospital."

"I've called for the ambulance—they're coming. We're out in the country and it takes time. I wanted you to know before she was taken to the hospital."

I began to formulate in my mind what could have caused her acute symptoms. Exacerbation of asthma with hypoxia was a possibility. Pleural effusion doesn't develop that suddenly. Or did she have a heart attack?

Then I realized I had forgotten to think of the most important condition, something hiding in plain sight—pulmonary embolism (PE), or blood clots in the lungs. A sudden onset of dyspnea, sweating, and tachycardia would all go along with PE. She was what we call in medicine "an ideal candidate" for embolism because of Tam. When the drug first began to be prescribed, we didn't think much of this side effect. But as Tam came into widespread use, more and more cases of thromboembolism were reported. Still, the rates were so low—about 1 percent—that in the larger context of battling cancer, it simply wasn't an everyday worry. Its benefits far outweighed its embolism risk.

But the favorable statistics hadn't favored Corina at all, for she had an obvious pulmonary embolism. Her symptoms quickly improved with oxygen and IV heparin, the standard anticoagulant. In a few days, she was asymptomatic and was sent home with warfarin, an oral blood thinner to prevent the recurrence of clots. She was to be monitored by her FP with a simple blood test called prothrombin time, a coagulation test that helps to adjust the warfarin dose. This is a tricky non-cancer drug if ever there was one: too high a dose could induce hemorrhage, while too low a dose could set off recurrent embolism.

Remembering warfarin's origin forces you to be cautious about its use. It's another drug that has a checkered history. First introduced as a rat poison in 1948, it ended up being one of the most useful agents in medicine since 1954. President Dwight Eisenhower was one of its early recipients, in 1955, after his heart attack.

Before Corina was discharged from the hospital, she brought up an issue that I hadn't settled.

"Do I restart Tam? It's been good to me all these years."

"Yes, at least as long as you are on the blood-thinning medicine. That will be for six months."

"Then what?"

"We can worry about it then."

The truth was that I wasn't sure what I would do after the six months passed.

"Can the lung clot come back if I take the Tam again?"

There was no definitive answer. But if Tam had caused the PE once, it could do this again despite the warfarin.

"It's a possibility," I acknowledged.

"It's a choice between having cancer or having a clot."

"That seems to be the case."

"Then I better follow your advice."

I hoped and prayed that my advice on restarting Tam was sound.

CHAPTER 8

About four months later, Corina came back to see me with severe pain in her lower back. She was now sixty-eight.

"I lifted a sack of grain a week ago," she said, "and that's when the pain started. Harold asked me not to lift anything heavy. But it's my old habit—if I can do something myself, I do it. I don't wait for him if he's busy on the farm."

Low back pain is one of those complaints that can throw you off balance. It's pervasive in our everyday lives, and it's not always easy to know what brought it on. Corina had a reason for the pain—she had lifted a heavy sack—but its persistence and severity bothered me.

"We better do a bone scan," I said.

"Can't you just give me some pain medicine and see if it'll go away? I had enough tests in the hospital four months ago."

"Pain medicine will relieve the pain, but it won't solve the problem. We need to find out what's causing it."

"Are you suspecting cancer?"

"I'm not sure."

"The last two times things turned out well, even though you were worried about cancer."

"You're right about that, but still, it's better to check."

The bone scan showed what's called hot spots, signs of metastasis, in the spine and hip. Had she run out of luck? Before we could determine that, another factor had to be considered. Tamoxifen itself can be responsible for the false-positive scan; because it heals metastatic lesions in bone, a follow-up scan may look different from before.

Corina's bone scan four months ago had showed "nonspecific" changes that didn't qualify as hot spots. When something looked vague in a scan or x-ray or didn't fit any specific diagnosis, the radiologists sometimes used the catch-all term "nonspecific." Could those nonspecific changes we saw before be metastases? If they were, we had missed them. The truth is that, even with all our technology, we can't find a cancer if it wants to remain hidden. The basic flaw of diagnosing cancer with scans and x-rays is this: tumors must be of a certain size before we can visualize them. That's the reason, as of now, annual mammograms are no longer recommended as routine for all women, only for those who meet certain criteria. Here's a sobering thought: because of the faulty notion about the power of machines, countless women have been put through small but cumulative doses of harmful radiation year after year.

When doctors encounter doubtful findings, they order additional tests. When we added all the pieces together, we came to an unfortunate conclusion: metastasis, not Tam, was the cause of Corina's hot spots. The tests also indicated that she had small lesions in her lungs.

I had to accept that Corina had developed resistance to Tam, like countless other patients had with chemo. I couldn't help having some recriminations. Had I compromised her treatment by stopping Tam during her PE? Cancer cells are always looking for a chance to re-attack their victims. Did I give them that chance? They are the masters of deception. After all, they were hiding in her body for decades, until they showed up in the pleura.

I told Corina what I had found. That the cancer was so widespread surprised her. "How is it possible," she asked, "to have so much cancer in four months?"

I explained the usual limitations in discovering a cancer in time.

"I was hoping my back pain was from a collapsed vertebra," she said, "and you'd give me good news as you did with the hip fracture and the abdominal lump."

"I wish I didn't have to give you the bad news."

"Looks like I don't have much time left?"

It's always hard to find a balance in answering a question like this—you want to express hope, yet not *false* hope.

"It's serious, but you've more time than you think. The twenty-six-year gap between the first diagnosis and first relapse is in your favor. And you responded well to the CMF and Tam. There's a fair chance of a treatment working again."

"What kind of treatment?"

"I'd like to give the CMF another try. It's been more than six years since you took it. The longer the interval between the chemos, the better the chance of a second success."

"At least I know what this chemo is. I didn't do too badly with it then."

I felt awful countering her confidence. "The chemo is the same, but the side effects could be greater. You have more cancer now, and you're weaker. And the character of a tumor changes with relapse, so it's hard to say how well you'll respond. Besides, we have another problem; currently, you're on a blood-thinner, so we have to watch out for bleeding."

She wasn't daunted by my explanation. "We'll do our best and pray," she said.

Corina managed to get through two cycles of CMF. After the third cycle, though, she had pneumonia. It took three weeks of antibiotics to clear the lung. By the time she felt well enough to take the next chemo, two months had gone by. Meanwhile, her back pain got worse, and her lesions increased. All this meant that the CMF had failed.

I needed to find another chemo for her. Doxorubicin (doxo), the anti-cancer antibiotic, was one of the most effective breast cancer drugs, but it exacted physical and other costs. Myelosuppression aside, severe nausea, vomiting, and fatigue could wear you down. But more serious was its lasting harm to the heart, leading to heart failure; the more you took, the higher the risks. That's why its cumulative dose had a limit, beyond which damage was irreversible.

As if this weren't enough, we also had to think of the hazards of administering doxo. Any extravasation, or leakage out of the vein into the surrounding tissues, caused blisters and cellulitis that could linger. Extravasations happened because of accidental displacement of the IV needle. In my training years, while doxo was still in one of its clinical trials, I had witnessed the aftermath of its tissue infiltration. Its potential for causing tissue damage made me forever extremely cautious when giving it. There's a safer way to inject it, however—through an indwelling venous catheter.

Because of its potential for causing mayhem (as well as its bright red color in solution) doxo had an unflattering moniker: the Red Devil. No one doubted doxo's anticancer power, Red Devil or not. But the acute nausea and vomiting during or immediately after its rapid infusion dispirited patients. It was, however, the standard method of infusion.

Corina was stoic, to be sure, but stoicism had its limits. I had doubts about whether she would be able to handle the prevailing method of injection. Luckily, a new, more tolerable technique had been introduced at MD Anderson and other centers. In this method, doxo was given in a continuous forty-eight-hour infusion through a small portable infusion pump; the pump was connected to an indwelling IV catheter, with the needle firmly secured. Patients went home with the pump, which was hidden under their garments. They and their family members were instructed ahead of time about the device. Those who had no family members to help were served by home health care nurses.

Corina, Cindy, and I went through our usual routine with a new treatment—what to expect and not to expect. Doxo's harsh side effects and the pump were our top concerns. The young woman cared for her mother-in-law a great deal and hoped for another remission. She encouraged Corina to accept the treatment and promised to take care of the pump. After some thought, Corina agreed.

Although she was of retirement age, she still continued to work part-time when she felt up to it. I had written to her employer to assign her a lighter duty, and her boss had taken her out of the kitchen and put her on the serving line in the cafeteria. Even then, I warned her about the limitations during this chemo, but she said, "Serving food to the kids in the cafeteria isn't hard."

In between her chemo, however, she sometimes became forgetful, though she didn't realize it herself. Schoolchildren can be mischievous. When she was at the lunch counter, a few of the kids discovered that she often lost track and devised ways to exploit her. They would go to her serving line several times to get multiple pieces of cake, which was against the school rules.

In the hustle and bustle of the hundreds of students dining at the same time, no coworker noticed the mischief. One afternoon, when the kitchen staff were doing inventory, a shortage of cakes was discovered. The boss was puzzled. He trusted Corina, who, he knew, certainly wouldn't pilfer anything. He decided to quietly watch the employees. To his surprise, he noticed that Corina had memory lapses. He caught the offending students.

Oncologists at first thought that this kind of forgetfulness was from the antiemetics and sedatives while on chemo. In fact, it's due to the so-called "chemo brain" or "chemo fog," a cognitive dysfunction that's an aftereffect of the chemo itself. But it's not yet well understood.

Interestingly, Corina's memory recovered after a few weeks. Still, would the foggy mind reappear with the next round of chemo?

CHAPTER 9

orina's back pain lessened after the first dose of doxo. In a responsive tumor, that's not uncommon—symptoms regress as the cancer regresses. Since side effects are less intense with the slow infusion compared to the rapid delivery, she managed to cope with the toxicity.

There's one more noxious part of being let down by the overly optimistic reports of new treatments. Even the most prestigious medical and scientific journals, which published papers on new treatments with fanfare from well-known academics and experts, have been forced to eat crow and retract their claims later. John Carlisle, a physician and medical sleuth, found numerous flawed and fraudulent clinical studies. General media, too, regularly report on the problem. Only when the researchers are caught are the studies withdrawn. But a lot of harm can be done before that happens, for it may take years to catch the deception.

Doxo and its slow infusion indeed proved beneficial. More gratifying news for Corina came after the third cycle: the bone metastasis had decreased, and the lung lesions weren't detectable. And, there was no chemo fog. Perhaps she didn't have it in the first place, and other factors played a part at the time.

With objective evidence of tumor shrinkage, we had reason to continue. Even though she had no cardiac symptoms to date, possible heart damage remained a concern. From the start, we had followed the protocol on checking her heart.

When the fourth dose was completed without incident, we were more optimistic than before, and we planned to give two more cycles, totaling six, and then do the follow-up evaluation again.

By the time the fifth treatment was due, however, Corina had developed palpitations, and her heart rate went from 80 to 120. The result of a repeat cardiac test was about the same as before.

While obsessing about chemotoxicity, doctors can get blindsided by the effects of nononcologic maladies. Another patient of mine on doxo, a thirty-two-year-old man with lymphoma, had tachycardia (rapid heart rate). His tachycardia, however, had nothing to do with the chemo. He was found to have thyrotoxicosis, in which the thyroid gland releases excess thyroid hormones into the circulation. Excess thyroid hormones stimulate the heart, and severe cases can result in heart failure. Fortunately, Corina's thyroid tests were normal.

I couldn't give Corina any more doxo without being sure about her heart, regardless of the tumor response. Also, widespread discussion about doxo's cardiac harm had overshadowed 5FU's rare potential for cardiotoxicity, which might have stressed her heart without symptoms when she received it with CMF twice in the past. Adding doxo had likely stressed it further, causing tachycardia.

I referred her to a cardiologist and told him what her treatments entailed.

The next day, he said, "The cardiac tests are okay."

"Something must be causing the tachycardia."

"I wish I could be more helpful."

At the time, cardiologists were still trying to figure out the nature of doxo cardiomyopathy (disease of the heart muscle). Serious heart damage from the drug can go up to 25 percent, depending on the age of the patient, the total dose, and concomitant other maladies.

I was looking for ways to continue doxo. The quality of Corina's life was still fair, and she had no symptoms from the tachycardia itself. The familiar quandary: if we stopped the drug now, the cancer would kill her. So far, she had received well below the total recommended dose of doxo. But could we rely solely on the cardiac tests as a guiding factor? Something hidden was going on, something that we had failed to put our fingers on. I couldn't get rid of the nagging disquiet inside me.

A year before, a woman in her fifties was referred to me from a Houston cancer center. She had metastatic breast cancer, and doxo put her into remission. A few months later, she became bedridden from refractory heart failure from cardiac damage. Her daughter brought her to San Angelo to nurse her in her last days. I hadn't forgotten the patient's pained expression as she told me, "I'm not dying of my cancer, I'm dying of its treatment."

All the precautions had been taken for her while she received the drug, including adhering to the cardiac protocol. In the end, the tests didn't save her. Chemo toxicities can occur anywhere, and it doesn't matter whether you are treated in Houston, Boston, New York, or San Angelo.

The unfortunate Houston woman taught me to be more cautious about Corina and remember that remission at any cost had no place in treatment. I decided to discontinue doxo. This wasn't the first surprise I had given her.

"Why? It's working," she said. "The heart doctor didn't find anything wrong, and the palpitations don't bother me."

"It's better to be cautious. More doxo can do permanent damage to your heart."

I had another reason for my decision to stop the chemo. A new hormone, megestrol, a synthetic progestin (the same hormone that's used alone or in combination in birth control) had been approved for metastatic breast cancer. It had already been on the market for treating cancer of the uterus.

Megestrol was perhaps the least harmful among the anticancer drugs. It didn't cause any nausea or vomiting; in fact, it had antiemetic properties. Moreover, as good as the hormone Tamoxifen was, some patients were beset by hot flashes. In contrast, megestrol was actually used to treat hot flashes in postmenopausal women. Besides, it wouldn't hurt the heart. True, it didn't have the power of doxo to abate a tumor, but it made up for that with its "benignity." Also, it could be easily taken in tablet or liquid form.

Corina couldn't have been more pleased with megestrol.

"It's different from the other treatments," she said after three weeks. "I had some anorexia left after the last chemo. It's gone now. I'm eating more and I've gained weight. I must be responding quickly."

I wished she were right, but hormones, unlike chemo, don't work that fast. Still, megestrol was special among the anticancer drugs: it offers another side benefit instead of another side effect—it stimulates appetite. That's why it's used in higher doses for the wasting syndrome in cancer and AIDS.

Corina's palpitations were gone in a few months. Perhaps it was because she was beyond doxo's surreptitious tricks. She again found a balance in her living.

CHAPTER 10

C orina had sinus congestion and headache off and on, and antihistamines relieved them. About a year after being on megestrol, she had them again. She did what she had done before—take antihistamines. But while the sinus congestion resolved, the headache got worse, and she felt weak and lethargic. She then came to see me.

She seemed uncharacteristically anxious.

"Anything else bothering you?" I asked.

"I fret a lot these days," she said. "Harold thinks that's not like me."

I examined her. She had a slightly unsteady gait, but that could be explained by her weakness. There were no other obvious neurological findings. Still, things didn't feel quite right.

"We should do a brain scan," I said.

"You did a CT of my head when I had a bad headache a few months ago, and you only found sinusitis. Antibiotics took care of that. That's what I need."

"You weren't weak then."

"Chemo makes me weak, too."

"Your last chemo was about a year ago."

She had also been reluctant to have a brain scan before. As sensible as she was, her reaction was understandable. Cancer patients accept myriad scans for treatments and follow-ups. A brain scan, however, has a different implication. Cancer is frightening enough in itself, but brain cancer incites more dread than most other kinds.

Corina accepted my reasoning, and I went ahead and ordered the CT.

I was no more eager than Corina to find brain metastasis. What she and I wanted, however, didn't matter to the CT. Though the cancer hadn't gone

99

to her brain itself, it had spread to its meninges. Meninges are the three layers of membranes—protective sheaths—that shield the brain and spinal cord. And within these layers, there is cerebrospinal fluid (CSF), a clear, colorless liquid that functions as a shock absorber.

When malignancy spreads to the meninges, it can induce carcinomatous meningitis. This is similar to bacterial or viral meningitis, in which the organisms inflame the meninges, bringing on acute symptoms of fever, intense headache, stiff neck, and visual disturbances. In carcinomatous meningitis, however, the symptoms aren't acute, and fever is absent, as it was for Corina.

But an x-ray abnormality isn't enough to diagnose meningeal cancer. We must have pathological proof and actually see the malignant cells under the microscope. It's akin to feeling a breast lump and then having a mammogram to confirm it. We still have to biopsy the lump to determine if it's malignant. But how do you prove a meningeal malignancy? Performing a biopsy would require opening the skull and resecting a piece of the meninges, a major surgery. Thankfully, we could avoid that procedure. The malignant cells from the meningeal membranes are shed in the CSF, so sampling this fluid and looking for the cells would give the answer. This was like checking her pleural fluid to find breast cancer cells when her pleural metastasis had been diagnosed years before.

Since the CSF surrounds the brain and spinal cord, it can be safely obtained by lumbar puncture (LP): inserting a hollow needle into the space between two lumbar vertebrae, then withdrawing several ccs of the fluid for microscopic study. It's an office procedure that I had done many times in my training and practicing years.

I told Corina about the lumbar puncture.

"I wish things were simpler with me," she said. But she agreed to the test.

The LP was performed. The report said there were no malignant cells. We oncologists love to hear "no malignant cells" in any report. Even then, we sometimes take this kind of report with caution. Why?

Unlike a lump biopsy, a CSF analysis can be treacherous. If enough cancer cells weren't yet shed into the fluid, they couldn't be detected easily. One negative report could give us false assurance, and all the while, the cancer would be growing in the meninges. Up to three lumbar punctures may be necessary to avoid this trap and confirm or refute the diagnosis.

It's a sensitive matter when you ask a patient to repeat a test for one reason or another, such as failing to make a diagnosis at the first try or getting a questionable result. But while it's one thing to repeat a chest x-ray, for example, it's quite another to redo an invasive procedure like LP. Patients may wonder about your acumen as a doctor or the quality of your lab, even though this happens everywhere, including at large cancer centers. Cancer, in its capriciousness, can make any doctor humble, vaunted or not.

I had to frustrate Corina again. During the second LP, I took out more fluid than before, hoping this would have more of the suspected cells and give us a better chance to find them. Withdrawing the CSF, however, requires delicate judgment. CSF volume and pressure rise with infection or cancer, the reason for the headache. Reducing the volume would reduce the pressure and relieve the headache. But taking out too much would lower the pressure unduly and imbalance the system, leading to unintended consequences: the low pressure, like the high pressure, would also provoke a headache. My second LP, therefore, temporarily worsened her symptoms, until the brain was able to manufacture more CSF to normalize the volume. It's similar to sudden swings in blood pressure; both too high and too low bring on symptoms.

This time the diagnosis was proven. I felt a mixture of apprehension and relief. Apprehension, because most patients with meningeal cancer died within six months—worse than her metastasis before. Relief, because I had no need to do a third LP. The more invasive procedures you do, the more chances of causing injury. This is called "iatrogenic" harm—harm induced by tests, treatments, or doctors.

I told Corina and Cindy what we were facing and the possible prognosis without treatment; and often, the treatment didn't work as well as it did with pleural metastasis. I added that meningeal cancer from breast was treatable, with occasional long survival. However, the treatment was more cumbersome than usual—especially for her because of the distance she had to travel.

Corina didn't surprise me—she took the news with equanimity. Cindy had a harder time. I advised Corina and Cindy to think about the therapy carefully.

The American Cancer Society, for which I was then a voluntary district director, and I had urged several San Angelo hotels to give discounted rates to patients like Corina, who couldn't get chemo or radiation without staying in town while on treatment. And the hotels had been kind enough to accommodate them. But that didn't solve all the problems, because for the safety of the patients, someone needed to stay with them. For working patients and family members, these kinds of treatments required more than usual jockeying and sacrifice. Cindy had a job as a secretary, and like other young mothers, she had small children or children in school.

I needed time, too, to think more. With Corina's likely short survival, how much was I willing to put her through?

Corina and Cindy came back with a decision.

"No one lives forever," Corina said. "I don't mind stopping here. I've lived long enough with cancer." Then she looked at Cindy and said, "But Cindy, Harold, and our children want me to give it another try. I'll do it for them."

Corina wasn't a weak-minded person by any means. I could understand her love for her family and their love for her, and for their sake, she would go the extra mile. She had been that way all her life.

There was no definitive guideline for treating her kind of cancer except that chemo was the main treatment, and methotrexate (MTX) was the drug of choice. There was a catch—for meningeal cancer, it had to be injected directly into the cerebrospinal fluid, a procedure known as intrathecal treatment (IT). To reach the CSF, you have to go through the meningeal membranes, or theca, that sheaths the spinal cord. The CSF volume being small—just 125 to 150 ccs—an IT allows the drug to saturate the meninges and potentially kill the cancer cells. Why not give oral, IV, or IM like other regimens? Because of a biological barrier to the brain called the blood-brain barrier, which prevents harmful substances from our circulation reaching our brain; these include bacteria, most chemo drugs, and medications. Hence, for meningeal treatment, IT is necessary to circumvent the barrier. Without this barrier, our brain would be damaged by many drugs and chemicals we take.

The IT can be administered through lumbar puncture, as for the CSF test. But the LP method has one practical disadvantage—one has to give MTX frequently, like twice-weekly to weekly to monthly, then at lesser intervals for months. All this means that you need to do dozens of LPs, which require piercing the lumbar region again and again. The law of averages dictates that no matter how good you are, on rare occasions, you have a chance of causing iatrogenic injuries.

IT gained prominence because it became an integral part of treatment for acute lymphoblastic leukemia (ALL), which has a propensity for infiltrating the meninges. Though ALL can occur in adults, it's mainly a childhood malignancy, and prophylactic IT chemo has led to its long remission and cure (in contrast to meningeal cancer). So it was necessary to have an IT mechanism that was less traumatic to children.

Luckily, one of the most brilliant pioneering neurosurgeons in the world, Ayub Khan Ommaya (1930–2008), came to the rescue and vastly simplified IT administration. He invented, among other things, the Ommaya reservoir. It's a mushroom-shaped, self-sealing silicone dome with a catheter. A small hole is drilled into the skull, and then the catheter is placed in the CSF ventricles inside the brain. The dome itself is placed just under the scalp and is easily seen and felt. Chemotherapy is injected through this dome to reach the CSF as often as needed, with little risk or discomfort. It's like injecting a drug through an indwelling IV catheter. The Ommaya reservoir is a highly effective implant. It allows easy, long-term access to the cerebrospinal fluid to deliver not only chemo but also antimicrobials directly into the brain. It has been a lifesaver for children with ALL.

Corina accepted the Ommaya, and after it was inserted, we started the IT-MTX protocol. She handled the treatment well. Once, though, she commented on her current life with a tone of regret.

"I've enjoyed my work at the school," she said, "but I'm not much use anymore. My bosses also know that, but they still keep telling me I'm needed, and I'm welcome to come back anytime I can. Yes, I have my husband, children, and grandchildren. They're with me because I'm theirs, they have no choice. My school had a choice to cut me off, but they've kept me this long." Then she added something that she hadn't said directly before: "God has a hand in everything."

I had felt all along that Corina was religious, but she had kept it quiet. I have seen the likes of her whose faith and spirituality stay inside them, without an outward display. For many, the belief that a higher power is watching over them gives them strength to duel with the travails of life. My grandmother was one of them. She had been through more than her share of heartbreaks—the deaths of her husband at a young age (before I was born), of her first son, and her beloved daughter-in-law, my mother. All she said was, "It's God's will." And through all this, my grandmother raised and guided her family and supported others in their hard times. Even in that male-dominated culture, the poor leaned on her.

In my practice, I had always appreciated the kindness of clerics—among them were ministers and priests—some of whom were my friends; they helped quite a few of my patients, especially the poor, to cope with their darkest days.

Besides injecting chemo into the Ommaya, the reservoir also allowed CSF to be easily drawn through it to do the follow-up tests. In a few weeks, the malignant cells were gone from Corina's CSF. But to eradicate the possible hidden cancer in the meninges, the IT chemo had to be continued for months.

About five months later, Corina caught the flu, even though she had received adequate flu vaccines. Her immunity was breaking down more. Viral infections, unlike most bacterial infections, can have an odd effect on the blood. They can suppress the bone marrow, causing pancytopenia—the simultaneous depression of red cells, white cells, and platelets, meaning that it is a more serious form of myelosuppression. That's what happened to Corina. Her platelets dropped so low that she lost a lot of blood from nosebleeds. I was hoping her myelosuppression was due to viremia, not MTX, and that it was temporary since it resolved when the viremia resolved. I had treated patients with this kind of viremic pancytopenia quite a few times.

However, the pancytopenia progressed even after Corina recovered from the flu. I realized that her bone marrow had quietly transformed for the worse; it had mutated with time. As a part of the CMF chemo years ago, she had received a leukemogenic drug, cyclophosphamide. That drug had induced myelodysplastic syndrome (MDS), an incurable preleukemic condition. The flu happened to make the weak bone marrow weaker and bring the MDS into the open.

We were dealing with another painful irony that I saw in the Houston woman who died of doxo. Corina's fate, similarly, wasn't decided by her breast cancer, but by all the mutagenic chemo I had prescribed. The treatments had prolonged her life, but she was paying dearly for that privilege.

This paradox wasn't easy to reconcile. At Dhaka Medical College Hospital, many of our cancer patients died from inadequate therapy due to a lack of resources. But in the United States, some of our patients die from our most sophisticated treatments.

"How much should I do for Corina now?" I asked myself, as if I were asking the question of someone else. Not much, really, was the answer. All I could do was keep her comfortable with palliative care. She, too, was ready for that.

It was hard for me to give up my long bond with her. She was someone with a rare strength to console others, including me, even in the midst of her trying times. I checked my feeling of loss before I let go of her for the final time. I didn't realize it would be so difficult. I had said farewell to her many times after her chemos, knowing that she would be back for the next treatment. But this time she wouldn't be back. She must have seen my pained expression.

"You shouldn't feel bad," she said. "You've tried. I've made it nine years since you first saw me. Most people don't live this long after their cancer has spread this much. Don't forget, I've had this cancer for thirty-five years."

I owed Corina Johnson a great deal. She gave me the impetus to try the slow infusion of a two-drug combination, doxorubicin plus vinblastine, on women of seventy-five-plus years. The treatment successfully controlled their metastatic breast cancer for a significant period. Later, I presented my experience, limited as it was, at a national breast cancer symposium in San Antonio, and then published it as an abstract in the 1985 *Proceedings of the American Society of Clinical Oncology*.

I wanted to refer Corina to a hospice, but a nurse friend of hers, Maria Ramirez, had opened a home health care service in a small country town close to her home.

"Corina has been very good to me all my life," Maria said, "even when she was sick. I was about fourteen when my mother died. I had a hard time losing her, and things got worse when my father remarried two years later. Corina took me under her wing. I would've run away from home if she hadn't been there. God knows what would've happened to me without her. She has also helped so many others, I know. Please give me a chance to give something back to her."

"It's terminal care," I cautioned. "Medicare may not reimburse home health service for her."

"It doesn't matter to me."

"She may linger longer than you think, and palliative care can be time-consuming."

"I want her to be with me as long as possible. I know I'm not hospice, but I promise to do my best."

I agreed. Corina herself was pleased with this arrangement. Maria kept her word; she did everything possible to keep her friend and patient comfortable. Seven weeks later, Corina died peacefully.

Whenever I am flustered by a setback, I try to think of Corina to reorient myself. Equanimity can soften the impact of a blow. I often remember how she sacrificed for others—giving herself and her time to them. It is truly a sacrifice when your days are numbered and time is your most precious possession.

I was heartened by the fact that her kindness was returned in some measure by Maria Ramirez. Maria, too, was a light—she showed us the meaning of gratitude, the meaning that many of us often forget.

But there is more to Corina Johnson's story. She made me reflect on the dangers of dogma in medicine. Cruel, disfiguring radical mastectomy, which caused so much suffering for women, was an unshakable dogma for decades. Then, a few brave surgeons challenged that hidebound tradition and abandoned it. That's how we arrived at less and less invasive surgery—from modified radical mastectomy to simple mastectomy to just lumpectomy. Recently, a preliminary study, led by MD Anderson Cancer Center, has shown that for some early breast cancers, surgery may not be needed at all; a short course of chemo with radiation would be enough to achieve remission. But even if it's confirmed with larger and longer studies, this newer plan of treatment may still look too invasive as we learn more—who knows? As science, technology, and procedures evolve, I am reminded that dogma has no place in medicine and science.

PART 3

J. D.:
MONEY OR LIFE?

CHAPTER 11

J ames Davis (J. D.), a robust forty-six-year-old man, developed blurred vision in his left eye without warning. He thought he'd had a stroke of some kind, for when his elderly aunt suffered a mild stroke not too long before, she had a similar eye problem.

His primary physician didn't find any neurological problems, and there was nothing wrong with his right eye. An MRI of his brain was normal. J. D. was sent to an ophthalmologist, Dr. M. It was Dr. M who referred J. D. to me.

"I can't quite get a handle on it," Dr. M said to me, "but there's something fishy here. I think I see a tiny fleck in the retina of his blurred eye. He has a slightly high white cell count. I don't know if it has any connection to this; maybe I'm reading too much into it. Would you see J. D. to make sense of his blood count?"

J. D. looked like the picture of health to me. He was a muscular, big-boned man and had no other symptoms or signs except the blurred vision. He was active and working as a foreman of a huge ranch.

Oncologists are always conscious of possible laboratory errors. I repeated his CBC—complete blood count—in our own clinic to make sure his first report was correct. It was.

I then looked at his blood slides under the microscope. He did have a few more bands than usual; bands are a type of mildly immature neutrophils, the type of white cells that fight infection.

After the blood cells are produced in the bone marrow, they go through different stages of growth to become mature. Normally, the cells migrate from the marrow to the circulating blood only in mature form. The immature types, however, can show up in the blood—sometimes called shift to the left—in response to diseases or conditions such as infection or inflammation. J. D.

had no sign of infection, however. Inflammation, though, can be induced by trauma, among other things. Since a ranch worker often works with heavy machinery, I asked him if he had any recent injuries.

"I didn't have any injuries," he said, "but I did have sinus infection. You know how dusty West Texas is without rain. You can't avoid inhaling the dust when you work on a farm or ranch. But it's been three weeks since the infection; amoxicillin cleared it up. My eye problem started five days ago."

His white blood cell (WBC) count was only slightly higher than normal, 12,000 (normal being 4,500 to 11,000). He had no other blood problem. So I thought the mild changes in his white cells were self-limiting phenomena that had nothing to do with his visual anomaly. Therefore, I could follow his labs and let Dr. M follow the eye abnormality to see if it would return to normal on its own. The idea sounded reasonable until I mulled over the retinal fleck. Dr. M was a perceptive physician, and I took his suspicions seriously. If the fleck were real, J. D. could have something serious. But in a healthy, active ranch man, it wouldn't be easy to broach this possibility. If I were wrong, I would have made a mountain out of a molehill, and he wouldn't look at me kindly. The more I thought of the retinal lesion, however, the more it bothered me. I decided to face the issue head on.

"Your blood count may be due to a leukemoid reaction to something," I said to him. "It's called leukemoid because it looks like leukemia, but it's not. I can't find any obvious reason for this. We should do more tests to verify what it is."

Actually, a form of leukemia was in my mind, but I put the news to him this way to soften my approach.

"How do you make sure?" he asked.

"With a blood test called BCR-ABL. It separates the leukemoid reaction from chronic myeloid leukemia, commonly called CML, one of the many leukemias."

He was startled. "Dr. M said I had a minor blood problem. Leukemia is bad!"

"You're right. But once in a while, leukemia cells can settle in the retina. The BCR-ABL can help us to rule out leukemia."

He shook his head. "Dr. M didn't even give me a hint of leukemia."

"But he had a reason for referring you to me. The retinal fleck and the white cells concerned him enough."

J. D. was still baffled, but he agreed to the test.

BCR-ABL is an oncogene. Oncogenes are mutated genes that have the potential to cause cancer. The BCR-ABL itself transforms normal white blood cells into leukemic cells.

Each cell in our body has twenty-three pairs of numbered chromosomes, which contain our genes. Normally, they work like clockwork to maintain our cellular functions without our knowing. But in CML, this inner machinery goes haywire, and the structure of two of the chromosomes—numbers nine and twenty-two—are altered. A piece of chromosome nine and a piece of chromosome twenty-two break off and trade places, creating a fusion gene on chromosome twenty-two. This fusion gene is the oncogene BCR-ABL. The altered chromosome twenty-two with this abnormal gene is known as the Philadelphia chromosome, or Ph chromosome, because it was discovered in Philadelphia in 1959 by David Hungerford and Peter Nowell. Before their discovery, there was widespread skepticism that genetic changes could induce cancer. These two scientists forever changed our thinking on a fundamental factor in cancer.

The BCR-ABL test, a molecular test, was devised to diagnose and follow chronic myeloid leukemia. It's an extremely sensitive test and helps to detect CML at its earliest stage, at the molecular level, before its more obvious signs show up in the blood.

Oncologists live on hope, and depending on what they are dealing with, they hope for either a positive or a negative result after ordering a test. For example, in breast cancer, positive estrogen and progesterone receptors in malignant cells signal a good prognosis, while negative receptors suggest a poorer outcome. With BCR-ABL, its presence would signify leukemia. The hope for J. D. was a negative result.

Although I subscribed to hope, I knew about life; sometimes hope alone may not give you what you want. J. D.'s BCR-ABL was positive, which meant that his white cells had the Ph chromosome. Taking everything together, the diagnosis was conclusively CML. There was a silver lining, though: those with the presence of the Ph chromosome in the cells live longer than those without. (All CMLs have abnormal cellular changes, but in a small group, the Philadelphia chromosome is absent, indicating a poorer prognosis. These cases are diagnosed from other hematologic aberrations.)

"J. D.," I said, "I'm afraid you have chronic myeloid leukemia."

"That's hard to believe," he said sharply. "I don't feel sick. Doesn't leukemia make you sick?"

"The acute leukemias are the kinds that are aggressive from the start and can make you sick quickly. But the chronic leukemias are slow growing, and you may not have any symptoms for a long time."

Since leukemia, like myeloma, starts in the bone marrow, taking a BM sample and looking at it under the microscope is routine for the diagnosis. Moreover, analysis of the Ph chromosome is done in the bone marrow cells. The BCR-ABL test itself, however, can be performed with a small blood sample.

"How did the leukemia get into my eye?" J. D. asked.

"Leukemia cells from the bone marrow circulate in the blood, and like any cancer, they can settle in any organ or place. Yours is a bit unusual in that it went to the retina first. If it hadn't, you might have waited until it progressed."

"You mean my blurred vision helped?"

"In a way, yes. Dr. M actually caught it early. If he waited until the retinal lesion was obvious, the leukemia would've been worse."

"Since my eye is the problem now, what can we do about it?"

"Once we control the CML, the eye infiltrate will clear up, and the blurring will go away."

"Do I need chemotherapy? I know chemotherapy is hard on people."

"I don't want any cancer for myself, but if I had to have one, I'd rather have CML. We have a new breakthrough drug called imatinib. It's not chemotherapy, but it's very effective."

"I've read about a lot of cancer breakthroughs. So how come we still have so much cancer?"

J. D.'s doubt about "cancer breakthroughs" was understandable. He had kept up some with cancer news, as some people do. The term "breakthrough" is thrown around indiscriminately whenever a promising new cancer drug comes along. Interferon is a prime example. Its manufacturer spent countless millions to promote it among oncologists, touting it as a natural substance, a nontoxic agent, in contrast to chemo. Books and articles on interferon's virtues proliferated in the 1980s. *Time* magazine even had a catchy cover story on March 31, 1980, titled, "Interferon: the IF drug for cancer." Interferon had a cachet that others didn't—it was the first genetically engineered cancer drug to be commercially approved. Even politicians got in on the act. Otis R. Bowen, then the Secretary of Health and Human Services, said about interferon, "It marks a new age in medicine." No wonder that, in the public mind, it was deemed almost a cure-all.

I, too, was caught up in the excitement and took part in the promotion in my early career. Interferon's manufacturer invited hundreds of doctors from around the world, including me, to Bermuda, ostensibly for an educational symposium on the agent. Most of the attendees, however, were from the US. The symposium was led by a prominent academic oncologist from a prestigious cancer center. The participants stayed in a luxury hotel, and all the expenses, including airfare, were paid for by the company. A great deal of time at the meetings was spent hyping interferon, and the rest for the entertainment of the doctors. Indeed, it was educational for me in more ways than one. What I learned in Bermuda could easily have been learned sitting in Texas, and cheaply. Once I caught on to the gimmicks, I refused to take part in such an event again. Unfortunately, at the time, this kind of lavish promotion was also offered by other drugmakers. Patients, of course, paid for these huge costs with high drug prices.

Alas, for cancer patients, interferon didn't turn out the way it was supposed to. Except for hairy cell leukemia, a rare disease, and for some CML and melanoma, it didn't work in most malignancies. Considering its cost and toxicity—and it's surely a toxic agent—it had only limited success. This was another hard lesson for me on the subject of drug promotion.

Because of this kind of unwarranted publicity, when a real breakthrough that changes patient care is discovered, it takes time for the public to believe in it. Imatinib is one of those drugs that deserves to be called revolutionary. It was invented in the late 1990s by the biochemist Nicholas Lydon. The brainchild for its use in CML, however, belonged to Brian Druker at the Dana-Farber Cancer Institute. He and his group, and Hagop Kantarjian and his colleagues at MD Anderson Cancer Center, among others, spearheaded clinical trials that led to the FDA approval of imatinib in 2001.

I remember how unsatisfactory CML treatment was before imatinib arrived. We used two old drugs, hydroxyurea and busulfan. These are tablets that are easy to take and cause little nausea. Although they had their benefits, they also had marked limitations.

In CML, the white cell count can go staggeringly high, up to 500,000 or more (normal is only 4,500 to 11,000). This large number of cells can clog blood vessels, leading to stroke and other complications, especially in older patients. Hydroxyurea could reduce the count to safer levels, but that's all it did. It had no power to induce remission.

Busulfan worked better to control CML, but with scant long-term benefit. On rare occasions, it caused a dangerous side effect, aplastic anemia, in which the bone marrow is severely damaged, leading to pancytopenia: anemia, low white cells and platelets. Every time I prescribed busulfan, I dreaded this pernicious effect. There was a reason for this.

In the early part of my practice, in the mid-1970s, one of my patients, a fifty-seven-year-old woman with CML, had "aplastic anemia" for months from busulfan treatment. She required multiple blood transfusions for anemia and antibiotics for infections due to markedly low white cells; she also had nosebleeds and extensive bruises from the low platelets. These complications required several rounds of prolonged hospitalizations.

I planned to send her for a bone marrow transplant, a desperate procedure for both aplastic anemia and CML. I was trying to find a marrow donor among her siblings scattered around the country. These things took time to arrange, and while we were doing all this, her white cells began to improve slowly. Eventually, her CBC became normal. What she really had was protracted but reversible myelosuppression, not irreversible aplastic anemia. I was relieved.

That relief didn't last long. Once the busulfan effect was gone, her leukemia rose again. This time, she was sicker than before and refused to have the BMT. Since high-dose chemotherapy is part of the BMT, for good reason, she dreaded its life-threatening toxicities. "I'd rather die than be stuck in the hospital all the time," she said.

The leukemia granted her wish. Her CML transformed into acute leukemia, as CML does, and she died shortly after. I never forgot the tragedy and how I lost her.

No wonder that after busulfan and interferon, imatinib was a stroke of luck for patients. It permanently changed the lives of CML sufferers. Synthetically produced in tablet form, it was a completely new innovation, the first of its kind. It's how the drug kills cancer cells that makes it so appealing. The BCR-ABL oncogene induces CML by stimulating a protein called tyrosine kinase, which helps the leukemia cells multiply endlessly. Therefore, if you specifically target this kinase and inhibit it, you block the leukemia;

imatinib does that. This became known as targeted therapy. (The principle of targeted therapy is also described in part 1.) Once imatinib showed the way, a whole slew of kinase inhibitors came onto the market for CML and various other cancers, and this class of drugs became known as the tyrosine kinase inhibitors or TKIs.

It's not that imatinib was entirely benign. It caused myelosuppression, edema, nausea, and other toxicities. But for the vast majority of cancer sufferers, it was nowhere near as onerous as chemo drugs.

J. D. began Gleevec, the brand name for imatinib, as soon as his insurance approved it. Its dose is 400–800 mg daily, and he got the lower dose because his leukemia was in the early phase. I strongly anticipated that he would go into remission quickly since his WBC was only slightly high, just 12,000.

A few weeks into the treatment, J. D. confided to me with a tone of gratitude, "Your medicine has really worked. My blurry vision is gone."

Sally, his wife, often came with him during treatments. She spoke more freely than he did.

"Thank you for helping him," she said. "He was miserable because he was unsure about his job. It's a big ranch, with a lot of cattle to supervise and a lot of fences to build. The ranch also has a lot of oil wells. He has to watch the drillers—you know how some drillers can damage the land. I can tell his eye is better because he's back to his stubborn self."

Dr M, the referring ophthalmologist, also talked to me about J. D. "Remember his retinal lesion I told you about? It's gone. It was a leukemic infiltrate after all. He's told me about Gleevec. I didn't know much about it, so I read up on it." Then he ruefully added, "I wish we had a Gleevec in ophthalmology. Vision loss from macular degeneration is hard to deal with, but we don't have a drug like that for something so common."

Oncologists get thanks from our patients even when the latter are doing poorly. But it's not too often that we get this kind of compliment simultaneously from our colleagues as well as our patients and their families.

CML responds to TKIs like Gleevec in three stages: from reverting to normal WBC to the disappearance of the Ph chromosome to the elimination of the BCR-ABL oncogene. The total elimination of the oncogene, the most desired outcome, is called the complete molecular response (CMR), and it may take months.

J. D.'s WBC became normal in a few weeks, so he had achieved the first leg of the response, a harbinger of good news ahead. In a few months, the Ph chromosome vanished from the leukemia cells. Then a year or so later, he achieved the hoped-for CMR. We were sure his leukemia was gone.

"I can't thank you enough . . . Dr. R," J. D. choked back tears. For a reserved man, that was a lot. Sally held me in a hug and stayed quiet.

Although Gleevec was a superdrug, it wasn't a magic potion. It had to be continued for an indefinite period to sustain the remission, like taking daily medicine for blood pressure. That was the thinking in 2003 when J. D. was diagnosed.

He continued the drug as I advised. Nausea was the main problem, but a new, expensive antinausea medicine, Zofran, took care of that. So CML and its treatment didn't limit J. D. Then, he encountered a setback that he couldn't have foreseen.

CHAPTER 12

D octors often forget that cancer patients face the same difficulties that the rest of us do; they have to carry the burdens of cancer along with the other burdens of living. At times, the non-cancer burdens can be heavier than the cancer itself. That's what happened to J. D. when a big agricultural company bought his ranch.

"The new company wanted to consolidate the operation," J. D. said. "That's an excuse to lay off employees, even though my ranch was making a good profit."

He was a dedicated worker and had received commendations and promotions over the years, so he thought his own job was secure—but he was wrong.

"I never thought I'd get axed," he said. "Maybe it was because of my salary. They could've cut down my salary and kept me. Twenty-six years I've been working for them. I started as a helping hand, then worked my way up to supervising foreman. Once I was a foreman, I worked more than the others, without overtime pay. What good did it do me?"

The whole of West Texas depends on ranching, farming, and oil. They are connected to each other in the economic sphere, and they all need employees willing to do the necessary backbreaking labor. When oil prices soar, the drilling business mushrooms, and they can't find enough employees. But when the price collapses, some drillers go bankrupt, and their jobs vanish. In between, if the giants swallow their rivals, big or small, employees are left in the lurch.

Oil booms and busts are regular features in Texas life, as are the ordinary high and low prices. When J. D. lost his ranch job, it was a period of low. A small, shady oil driller who began at the high was plagued by accidents—he cut corners on safety to make a quick killing. With the low oil prices, he was about to go under when a new owner bought him out at a bargain price.

The new owner tried to make it work, but it was harder than he thought because of the company's past reputation. J. D. had some experience in oil work from his ranching days, and he had a knack for training workers and solving mechanical problems. The new owner liked him and gave him a chance by offering him a new job. It wasn't long before he turned the company's safety record around.

"Saving the company made me happy," he said. "It's prevented quite a few layoffs. I know how it feels to be cast out."

For his new job, however, he had to live far away from home. I gave him a three-month Gleevec prescription. While on the drug, it's routine to do periodic CBC to make sure the treatment is working, but not suppressing the count too much. J. D. had done the CBC regularly so far, and it had been stable. But now he had a practical problem doing the blood counts.

"It's not easy to drive to a town from the oil fields in the sticks," he said. "And I can't waste money on gas with all the coming and going. Besides, I don't want to take off too much to get the blood tests. I started at the company recently, and I don't want to get fired again."

We made a compromise. He would come to see me in three months and have the CBC. If he had any problems before that, he would get the lab work done at the nearest clinic or hospital.

He didn't, however, keep his appointment with me or contact me for four months. Then one day, he came to see me with fever and weakness. I thought he had some kind of infection. But his CBC troubled me—his white cell count had gone up from a normal 5,000 the last time to 80,000. More worrisome, J. D. had many abnormal cells in his blood.

What did all this mean? The meaning was connected to the life of CML. In general, the evolution of the leukemia takes place in stages: from the chronic phase to the accelerated phase to the blastic phase.

Chronic phase: The chronic phase is a slow-growing state in which patients may or may not have symptoms.

Accelerated phase: In this phase, CML is accelerating, and patients have symptoms such as fever, fatigue, and night sweats and early satiety and abdominal pain if the spleen is enlarged.

Blastic phase or blast crisis: In the third phase, the disease has turned into acute leukemia. Blasts are the most immature form of bone marrow cells and are the most virulent when they are malignant. Hence, "blast crisis" is an appropriate term, because this transformation into acute leukemia is indeed a deadly crisis. The symptoms are more pronounced.

J. D.'s illness started with a leisurely chronic phase, with just a slightly high WBC count and no symptoms besides his blurred vision. But now it was different—his white cells were sixteen times higher than before, and he had fever and weakness, all from the leukemia. I feared he had developed resistance to Gleevec, like other cancer patients sometimes do with chemo. This was entirely unexpected, since he'd had such a good response and a smooth course before.

I had tried to keep the possibility of resistance out of my thoughts—I had so much faith in Gleevec. But now, it was what it was. I had to deliver the bad news again.

"I'm sorry, J. D., the CML is progressing faster now. That's why you have fever and fatigue. Your leukemia has become resistant to Gleevec. We may be able to overcome this by doubling the dose to 800 mg daily. But the higher dose may also give you more side effects."

J. D. stayed silent, but Sally looked at him angrily and demanded, "How can you have resistance?"

"It happens with all medicines," I interjected gently, somewhat surprised by her anger.

"Since he saw you, Dr. R, he's been away from home," Sally added. "He hasn't taken Gleevec all this time. I didn't know anything about this until now. He keeps things to himself. It makes me mad."

I, too, was flabbergasted. How could that happen? He was a responsible, hard-working man, and I had accommodated him because of the vagaries of his work.

"What's going on, J. D.?" I asked.

He looked me straight in the eye and said, "Sally doesn't understand. I lost my health insurance when I lost my job. It took me a while to find work again. And I've got a long waiting period before the new insurance kicks in because I'm a high risk. I couldn't afford to spend $15,000 a month just on myself. I have to support her and our three children."

I was so enamored of Gleevec that I had neglected to consider its exorbitant cost. There are stratagems in drug pricing—the prices can vary according to where you are, what kind of health insurance you have, or whether you pay in cash. Mostly, the manufacturers and the middlemen decide how much they can get away with.

The starting dose of Gleevec for J. D.'s chronic phase CML was 400 mg daily, and to prevent nausea from it he had to take Zofran 8 mg twice a day. The cash price for a month of Gleevec was $12,000 and for Zofran $2,300. So, the total cost for these two drugs alone was $14,300 per month—that is, $477 a day. Then, in some months, labs, x-rays, and doctors' fees added about $1,000 more. At least when J. D. had insurance, it paid 80 percent and he paid 20 percent. Without insurance, he would have to pay the cash price from his own pocket, and the amount was far above his monthly income.

J. D.'s experience, like Clara Anderson's, starkly outlined an issue that plagues cancer victims—the crushing economic burdens of the newer drugs. These excesses had been going unchecked for a long time.

Surveying this regrettable state, in 2014, fully twenty-two years after my 1992 protest in the *New York Times* about abusive drug pricing, Hagop Kantarjian of MD Anderson Cancer Center gave a blunt warning to drug companies: "They are making the prices unreasonable, unsustainable, and, in my opinion, immoral." Kantarjian certainly knew what he was talking about—he had been a leader in leukemia research and treatment. Again, what good are superdrugs if their costs are out of reach for our patients?

A lot of cancer patients have gone bankrupt because of medical costs. One was Keneene Lewis, a thirty-nine-year-old woman with stage three out of four breast cancer. She had high-deductible insurance, which was all she could afford even with her two jobs. While struggling to get better with surgery, radiation, and chemo, she worked in between her treatments in her weakened condition and, at the same time, cared for her daughter as a single mother. Amidst all this, she was also fending off bill collectors. She was on the brink of becoming homeless and desperately managed to keep food on the table and a roof over their heads. She expressed the feeling of too many who are forced into dire straits: "Money is the last thing you should have to worry about when you are dealing with cancer and fighting for your life." The patients are simultaneously hit by malignancy as well as what's now called the "financial toxicity of cancer."

Moreover, other patients, with cancer or not, are also trapped by drug expenses. A recent CDC report on this should concern us all. In 2021, about 9.2 million adults, more than 8 percent of adults who are taking medications, tried to save money by waiting to fill a prescription, taking less than the prescribed dose, or skipping doses altogether. These measures have consequences, much like J. D.'s had in the end. The patients' diseases may worsen, and then more funds will be needed to manage their worse illnesses. In addition, besides their loss of productivity, the quality of their lives will be impaired.

With the leukemia back, I asked J. D. to start Gleevec as soon as possible.

J. D. looked at Sally, seeming hesitant about what to say. But Sally firmly told him, "You'll start it, even if I have to borrow or beg. I'll go back to my secretarial job I had before. I can ask my mother to help with the kids."

J. D. first wanted to try his original dose of Gleevec 400 mg daily before raising it. Of course, I hoped that this amount would still benefit him, but I wasn't sure if it would. If I tried to push the 800 mg, he might balk, and the atmosphere was already tense. Only time would settle these things.

I also asked for weekly CBC to monitor the response. Each time, I waited anxiously for the report. The WBC stayed stable for a while and then began to go up slowly. The Gleevec dose was increased. But his WBC kept fluctuating between 80,000 and 90,000. Though his fever went down, his BCR-ABL level rose. It seemed that the drug and the cancer were in a tenacious battle. Gleevec was trying to repel the malignant cells, and if it could force them into retreat, it could claim the victory. But if the cells broke through its defense, the CML would surely advance into the accelerated phase. Then, the inevitable blast crisis and almost imminent death.

About six weeks later, J. D.'s fever and night sweats intensified again, and he was much weaker; the higher Gleevec doses gave him persistent nausea, anorexia, and aches and pains all over his body. The tests proved it: the leukemia had gotten the upper hand, and Gleevec had lost. A bone marrow transplant (BMT) was the next option after the TKI failed. I had told him in the past about the possibility of BMT, though without much emphasis, because of my faith in Gleevec. This time, I was forthright.

"Gleevec isn't working anymore," I said to him.

"I can see that. What new treatment do you have?"

"Bone marrow transplant."

"I was hoping things wouldn't come to that."

"The longer we wait, the more the chances of a blast crisis. Once that happens, BMT will be riskier and much less effective."

"I don't know if I can handle it. I saw what happened to a friend who had a transplant."

"Every patient is different, and you may do better than your friend. Transplants in CML have been successful."

Sally intervened. "I can't let him die. We'll do whatever it takes, Dr. R. He has no excuse; he's covered by insurance now and his boss is nice."

Sally was talking about her husband's employer, a man who also believed in gratitude; he hadn't forgotten how J. D. had saved him from ruin. He gave J. D. a leave of absence and kept him on the company's group insurance.

For a BMT, we first had to find a matching bone marrow donor—that is, whose marrow type was that of J. D.'s—then send both him and the donor to a referral center. He wanted the BMT hospital closest to our town. That was San Antonio, though it was still 200 miles away—and in big cities, shorter distances don't mean anything if you are stuck in heavy traffic for hours.

"How do you find a matching bone marrow donor?" Sally asked.

"Start with his siblings."

"J. D. has one sister and three brothers."

"That's great," I said.

I thought J. D.'s having four siblings was a divine intervention to bring him good luck when he needed it most. Genetically, our odds were that one in four siblings was going to match. We proceeded with optimism. But things weren't as simple as I had envisioned. The sister who was most fond of him was in bad health, and even if she was a likely match, she couldn't help. Two other siblings were in excellent health, and we tested them. Unfortunately, they didn't match. Our hope lay in the last of the siblings, the youngest brother.

"Let's get your brother in the lab," I said to J. D. "He'll be our good luck."

"He and I don't get along," J. D. said. "To tell you the truth, Ron and I are more like enemies than brothers."

Seeing my surprise, he added, "It's a long story. Our father had a big piece of land right outside San Angelo. He gave it to three of us and excluded Ron. Father was angry with him for marrying a Mexican girl. I'm close to my father and I didn't oppose him. Ron has held that against me."

I couldn't help asking why the siblings couldn't share the land with him on their own.

"It's a private matter that I better not get into. I'd be ashamed of begging him for a favor. Anyway, I know he'd reject me out of hand. I don't want to be humiliated by him."

Sally glared at her husband.

"Ron is a better man than you think. You and your family make him look like a monster because he stands up for his wife. Why can't you be honest? All of you hate Elena. But she's a good person, a manager at Verizon. She's the primary breadwinner for her family, and I think that rankles your father. A Mexican American woman with a college degree and independence. And none of you has ever been to college."

Sally had waded into sensitive territory. I had, in the past, heard many White patients use the designation "Mexican" as a derogatory term, meant to demean their Hispanic neighbors. That Mexican Americans have been a part of Texas for generations, long before it was a state, didn't matter to them. They looked down upon a marriage between Whites and Hispanics. Ironically, some of the most bigoted Whites had settled in Texas much more recently than the Mexican people they complained about.

Sally, clearly the opposite of such bigots, continued her offensive.

"Your other brothers are divorced, and they married the White girls your father approved of. But Ron and Elena have a good marriage, and she has a good future as an executive. That's more than I can say about any of you."

Sally was also alluding to a shift in the social landscape. Through time, Mexican Americans had become more visible in the mostly White workforce. More to the point, Hispanics weren't just maids and laborers, or farm and ranch hands; both Hispanic men and women were also professionals, businesspeople, and held leadership positions. These advances were a far cry from what I had learned from the personal stories of two Hispanics with whom I was well acquainted.

One was a patient of mine, a man in his mid-eighties. "I was the first Hispanic policeman in my town," he said. "I could only arrest Hispanics, not Whites. If I found White lawbreakers, I had to call a White officer and wait until he came to arrest them. By that time, some criminals managed to get away, and there was nothing I could do. But I was blamed for their escape anyway. During my time, Hispanic officers were rare in Texas, and I was excluded from the inner circle of White officers. And having women officers was unthinkable, White or Hispanic."

Another story came from a Hispanic person who was a friend of mine. He was a top vice president of the old GTE Corporation, the largest independent telephone company during the days of the Bell System, now a part of Verizon.

"When I was a high school junior and senior," he said, "I cleaned the GTE offices and grounds in San Angelo to save money for college. My parents were poor. I was ambitious, and somehow I felt that after I finished college, I'd come back here as an executive. I shared that thought with some of the White employees. A few of them snickered, 'A Mexican janitor as a boss? That'll be the day.' But this made me more determined to prove myself, and here I am today."

Sally's comments about Elena and Ron and about the whole family didn't sit well with J. D.

"Do you have to bring up these things to Dr. R?" he asked in irritation. "Haven't we got enough of our own troubles?"

"All right," she said. "I'll call Elena. She's sensible and can convince Ron to help us out. She'll understand me—she has a husband."

CHAPTER 13

I waited with hope to hear from J. D. about his brother. A few days later, it was Sally who called me.

"I had a heart-to-heart talk with Elena and Ron," she said. "Elena pointedly asked her husband, 'What if I needed bone marrow and J. D. could give it? What would you do? Save my life, or keep holding your grudge?'"

Ron went to his doctor and gave blood for the HLA typing, the matching test. When I read the report, I gave a sigh of relief—he was a good match for J. D.

But there was still one more hurdle beyond our control. BMT was an expensive treatment, which health plans loved to deny. What if J. D.'s insurance did so? And no transplant program, then or now, would accept a patient unless payment was guaranteed in one form or another.

Throughout the decades of my practice, I had come to know this matter well: unlike medical professionals who care for patients, most insurance doctors and nurses are bureaucrats. Cloaked as "reviewers," they are actually gatekeepers hired for just one purpose—to maximize the company profits. Some of these bureaucrats are more informed than others. Worst are the ones who simply adhere to the rigid formulas they have set up themselves. They have no understanding that people don't get sick or well according to formulas. Just as human character varies, so do disease and recovery. That's why I felt lucky whenever I came across a knowledgeable gatekeeper.

I sent J. D.'s medical records to his insurance carrier. About two weeks later I received a call from one of their reviewers. "We need more documentation," he said.

"I've given you all the records," I replied.

"Is his transplant absolutely necessary?"

"Yes. It'll give him a chance for survival. BMT for CML isn't an iffy procedure. It's well established, you can look in the literature."

"I'll check on that."

In another ten days, the reviewer approved the BMT, but with a condition—I would have to submit updates until the BMT was done. Sometimes the reviewers would ask for the same records again and again, not just the updates; at times, I wondered if the gatekeepers bothered to read the documents at all. This all seemed like another tactic to delay any payment as long as possible.

I thought J. D. had cleared all of the barriers, but there was yet another snag.

"My leave has expired," he said. "I should go back to work part-time. At least help in the office. I feel weak and achy, but I can still do some planning. The company has been good to me. I don't want to push my luck and lose the job. I'll continue Gleevec two tablets daily, I promise. It may still do me some good."

"It doesn't make sense, J. D.," I reminded him. "You know it's extremely serious."

I offered to talk to the owner to see if J. D. could extend his leave. After some hesitation, he agreed to let me try.

"It's life or death for J. D.," I said to the owner. "He appreciates your kindness and loves your company. I can't promise, but I believe after his BMT he has a good chance of returning to some kind of work."

The owner's sympathy shone through. "J. D. helped to save my company. I'll do what I can from my end."

Meanwhile, the leukemia wasn't staying silent. J. D.'s WBC and BCR-ABL levels were rising. I wanted to do another bone marrow to see what phase he was in; as time passed, I was getting more and more worried. But he wanted a few days to settle his family matters.

That "few days" became a few weeks. J. D. was devoted to his father and had given him financial support for years—the old man had crippling arthritis and emphysema. But the father felt that the son whom he had loved so much had now betrayed him. He was upset that J. D. had taken the side of "disgraced" Ron, whose generosity in saving J. D.'s life didn't matter to him. J. D. wasted his precious time reconciling with his dad when his own life was at stake.

After this, I had a better understanding of what Albert Camus, the literary genius, meant about his philosophy of human behavior and absurdity. As a practicing physician, I could especially relate to his classic, *The Plague*: even in disease and death, each person reacts in his or her own way. During an epidemic of plague in the Algerian city of Oran, the victims were dying like flies, and there was a quarantine, which led to the shortage of daily necessities. While some businesses and people were busy fleecing the public, others put their lives on the line to save the victims.

The COVID-19 pandemic was a parallel to the plague in the book—it exposed our true nature. To save victims of COVID-19, doctors, nurses, first responders, and others risked their lives and the lives of their loved ones. Many made the ultimate sacrifice in the course of their service: they died from the COVID-19 virus they were fighting. One particular death hit close to home. A medical school friend of mine from Dhaka retired after practicing in New York City for about forty years. When COVID-19, in its early days, threw NYC into turmoil, and when there were no vaccines yet, he volunteered to care for COVID patients in a hospital. He never returned home. He contracted the virus, struggled for life in the ICU, then died a lonely death like thousands of others.

Amidst this tragedy everywhere, some people and businesses had no qualms about gouging the public, such as stealing money from COVID-19 funds or charging twenty dollars for a two-dollar mask.

When J. D. returned to me, he was worse off than before. His night sweats had become drenching, and he fatigued easily. His CBC mirrored his condition. He had many blasts in the blood—4 percent—that he hadn't had on his last visit. The blast count is the primary criterion for diagnosing the accelerated phase (AP) and blastic phase or acute leukemia (AL). Different groups—such as MD Anderson Cancer Center, the International Bone Marrow Registry, and the World Health Organization—have propagated different rules for these diagnoses.

Oncologists are caught in a dilemma about which group to follow. We can't waffle at the bedside. To diagnose and treat patients, we have to adhere to certain basic principles. I used a well-established international rule: the patient must have at least 10 percent blasts for AP and 30 percent blasts for AL, either in the blood or in the bone marrow.

That said, what to make of J. D.'s 4 percent? Was he in the AP? Though he didn't quite meet the minimum 10 percent criterion, I couldn't discount his symptoms. His bone marrow might confirm or refute the AP diagnosis. But what if it didn't? That's how cancer is at times: conundrums arise, and doctors and patients feel cornered.

Finally, the results from his latest bone marrow test came back. J. D. had at least 30 percent blasts—he had AL, the deadly blast crisis. There was no room for confusion: he met more than the minimum requirement for any of the groups. But as bad as his marrow was, there was a silver lining for him again. J. D.'s CML had turned into acute lymphoblastic leukemia, the childhood variety, which responds to chemo better than the expected adult variety, acute myeloid leukemia. Still, there was a twist—his acute leukemia, like his chronic one, was Ph chromosome positive, but here, its significance was the opposite. While the Ph chromosome in CML signifies a good prognosis, it means a bad one in ALL. (Since the introduction of the TKIs, however, the prognosis of this group is improving.)

But what a disappointment for J. D.. Looking at his blood, the worst I was expecting was the accelerated phase. When CML advances, it's supposed to proceed in an orderly fashion in phases. It gives you time to absorb the changes and plan the treatment. But CML, being a cancer, plays its share of deceits, and sometimes jumps from the chronic to the acute without warning, skipping the middle phase. This deceit was played on J. D., a tragedy that was entirely avoidable if he did not stop Gleevec. The man who could have enjoyed life in remission was now facing death. The days of his just taking some tablets—of Gleevec—were gone. The BMT was moot with J. D.'s move to the acute phase. The first step in the new plan was to control the acute leukemia with chemo, which is more complex than usual, a regimen that lasts two to three years. It can be daunting, yet most patients complete it successfully. It's briefly described here to help the reader appreciate the patients' bravery and stamina and to convey the dilemma the oncologists face in giving a long, drawn-out treatment. Also, I explain it here to caution against losing empathy, even after seeing the same persons and hearing the same complaints again and again.

The chemo program—the Larson regimen—contains nine drugs: Cytoxan, daunorubicin, vincristine, prednisone, L-asparaginase, ARA-C, 6-MP, dexamethasone, and 6-thioguanine. They are taken in various combinations via three routes: oral, intravenous, and intrathecal.

The drugs were administered in sequential steps known as induction, consolidation, and maintenance. There's one more step in between called central nervous system (CNS) prophylaxis. (The brain and the spinal cord together comprise the CNS.) This treatment method is like that of the meningeal metastasis in breast cancer, described in part 2, including the insertion and use of the Ommaya reservoir.

The most toxic of the group was daunorubicin, a cousin of the antibiotic doxorubicin; it's given at the beginning of the treatment for the induction of remission, the most intensive part of the regimen. However, the maintenance, the last step and the longest part of the program, was somewhat easier to take, and some patients were able to work during it.

J. D. seemed accepting of things as they stood and paid more attention to the treatment as best as he could. He hadn't forgotten that missing Gleevec had brought him to this state. Since he had started with me, two other patients with early CML had gone into remission with the drug. Cancer patients often talk to each other while they are waiting in the lobby or sitting for hours in the chemo room while getting their intravenous treatments.

J. D. was reluctant to complain to me in front of Sally. But he was sensible enough to bring her with him to listen to our discussions. Sometimes, the situation got prickly when she would try to speak for him and answer his questions. J. D. would then get irritated and counter her sharply. One day, I intervened.

I smiled at Sally and said, "He's the patient, he can talk for himself."

"But he doesn't tell you everything, Dr. R," she protested.

J. D. shot back, "I tell him what's important for me, not all my troubles in the world."

He had a hard time with the induction chemo, for induction for acute leukemias is always difficult to bear. Sally was sturdy as a rock, keeping calm in times of need and buoying him up.

I did a follow-up bone marrow test after the induction. At first, I felt the usual trepidation about looking at his slides under the lens. With all the rough times he had been through, what if we hadn't made any dents in his disease?

What excuse would I give him and Sally? I had seen enough induction failures.

I peered through the lens, fixed my eyes on the slides, and was heartened by what I saw. The leukemic blasts were less than 5 percent, in the normal range. But I wanted more proof before calling it a complete remission, or CR. I waited for the results of the two crucial tests on the cells—cytogenetics and immunophenotyping. When they arrived, they confirmed my microscopic findings; he was in CR again, and the Ph chromosome was absent. Then came the outcome of the most important test of all, the BCR-ABL: he had achieved the CMR of our dreams. I happily delivered the news to J. D. and Sally. He became somber and she burst into tears.

J. D. did better with the next step, the consolidation, since his bone marrow was healthier and recovered faster during the chemo cycles.

We had some consternation about how much to do for the CNS prophylaxis—after all, it wasn't a treatment for meningeal involvement, which he didn't have clinically, but presumably a preventive measure. In cancer care, some things aren't settled without dispute. Since ALL is primarily a childhood leukemia, most of the understanding about it had come from treating children. And for them, combined IT chemo and radiation in the brain was the standard. Some experts also subscribed to this approach for the adult ALL. But those who didn't felt that CSF chemo alone was sufficient, and safer, because the combined effect of the chemo and radiation on the adult brain could impair mental acuity. J. D. and I did talk about his odds of survival at the start of his ALL treatment. Though five-year survival was 90 percent in children, it was only about 25–40 percent in adults, depending on age. After taking this into account, and with a chance of dementia if we added radiation, we settled for just the IT therapy for the CNS prophylaxis.

With the IT therapy and the rest of his treatment, J. D. was getting tired of the chemo. Once, he asked me hesitantly, "Would it be safe to take a little break?"

I understood how he felt, but I couldn't give him any slack, not again. "I'm afraid it wouldn't be a good idea."

He bent his head and stayed silent.

CHAPTER 14

Hope and dread are a part of life for cancer patients, and despair is an intractable foe. Despair can creep in with this kind of protracted chemo that's physically and mentally demanding. I had cautioned both J. D. and Sally about this aspect of treatment, and I did what I could to sustain his motivation.

Vincristine is one of the IV drugs in the Larson regimen. During his treatment, J. D. developed vincristine peripheral neuropathy, with a shuffling gait. Vincristine had done its damage. It's one of the most commonly used anticancer drugs; it's the primary agent for remission of childhood leukemia and has immensely changed the fate of children with this deadly disease. It has a quality that we needed—it causes little myelosuppression and nausea. Still, being what it is—a chemo drug—it has to have a vice: dose-dependent neuropathy. Fortunately, the neuropathy, unless severe, slowly ameliorates after the drug is stopped. So as much as we wanted to continue the course, we could not, for we were afraid of causing irreversible damage. The usual painful quandary with chemo: you are forced to discontinue a drug even if it's doing good because of its insufferable toxicity. We continued the other maintenance drugs.

With the development of neuropathy, J. D. became discouraged again. Just about then, we were greeted by rare good news. A second-generation TKI—tyrosine kinase inhibitor—was approved by the FDA. This was nilotinib, a lifesaver for those who became resistant to imatinib. J. D. began the drug with high expectations. For the moment, we weren't thinking of BMT. This was a relief for us all.

Nilotinib (Tasigna) wasn't just another armament; it was more than that. It worked not only in the chronic phase but also in the blast crisis, at least for a while. But I couldn't forget one unpleasant fact—even with the new agent, the chances of relapse lingered. I harbored the hope that if this happened to J. D., some super-KI would come onto the market to save him, and with less toxicity and cost. For now, we had to buy time. On occasion, buying time is all we oncologists do. Meanwhile, if we were forced to do BMT, I prayed that by then it would be safer and cheaper.

The TKIs have brought up another oncologic dilemma: they have made the BMT decision harder than before. TKIs are less onerous than BMT, and they don't require searching for donors and haggling with insurance companies. But, being very expensive, TKIs aren't entirely benign. How could I forget why J. D. had stopped his Gleevec in the first place, even though it had put him into remission? And these drugs had to be taken for years, since no one was sure at the time how long to continue. The current encouraging news is welcome: some early-stage patients in long remission can discontinue it, but they must be monitored closely. Besides, we need long-term follow-up to confirm that the remission will remain without the TKIs. If not, in the end, the accumulated price of the TKIs may exceed the cost of a BMT.

The price of TKIs has the potential to drop when they turn generic, as Gleevec has done to some extent—unless, of course, Big Pharma exploits the system. Like all oncologists, I hope that as research and technology advance, TKI-like agents will flood the market for all kinds of cancers.

The chemo and nilotinib had kept J. D.'s ALL in remission. After three years, he had to move west, 120 miles away to Midland–Odessa, a major oil hub in Texas. Before he left, I referred him to an oncologist there. By then, his neuropathy had improved, and he was stronger.

A few weeks later, I got a call from Sally. J. D. had gone to an oil field to supervise drilling. As a rule, the air at the oil fields is pungent with pollution. In the dry, barren country of far West Texas, dust storms come and go. While J. D. was in the field, he was caught in a storm and couldn't avoid inhaling dust. He developed acute bronchitis and sinusitis with fever. Sally called his new oncologist the same day. According to Sally, he curtly told her, "He blew up a good remission once. Do you want him to blow up another?" The doctor was upset because he had advised his patient to work in the office only, not in the oil fields. He had read in the patient's records how J. D. relapsed after a remission, but the doctor didn't care to know why. Since J. D. was a recent patient, the oncologist had no rapport with him yet. He asked Sally to take her husband to the ER. J. D. disliked going to the ER, and he was used to my accommodation. But now, he had no choice.

He got the usual x-rays and labs and got the antibiotic he needed. He improved in about two weeks.

Sally took exception to the oncologist's manner. "Why did you send us to him?" she asked me. "He acted like my husband was irresponsible and worthless."

"Everyone has a bad day once in a while," I said, not wanting to speak ill of a colleague.

"Are you looking for an excuse for a colleague's behavior?" She was upset.

I tried to find a way out. "Give him one more chance. If you still don't like him, I will get you another oncologist."

J. D.'s cancer doctor had gone into practice years after I had started. Several of his patients had already come to me for second opinions. He was actually a good clinician, but he expected his patients to follow his orders as given.

An internist who had been referring patients to me from the oncologist's town for a long time said to me, "Our oncologist is new, he's getting his feet wet. Too rigid with his recommendations."

I understood what he was talking about. The oncologist was still following the rules ingrained in him from his training years. But I also knew that time and experience would soften him for sure, as they did me and as they do everyone else.

After my conversation with Sally, I mulled over what she had said about the doctor's conduct. She wasn't far from the truth. At times, our pride gets in the way of patients' welfare, creating conflict and hurting the fragile bond between doctors and patients. I wondered how many times I had fallen short when it came to this.

My advice to Sally worked out well. When J. D. went to his next appointment, the doctor apologized to them both. Most of us are good enough to make amends for our failings.

I got news from J. D. once in a while. He continued to stay in remission on nilotinib. When I last heard from him, he was doing well—eight and a half years since he first saw me. This was in spite of the relapse with the acute leukemia that could have easily snuffed out his life.

As the years passed, the increasing good luck of my patients with CML—as with myeloma and breast cancer—gratified me. Take J. D. and his cohorts. When I began my practice forty-nine years ago, the vast majority of them would have died in four years, and certainly within six months of the acute leukemia of the blast crisis. Twenty-five years later, TKIs changed the grim landscape. Many of those who go into remission with TKIs are expected to have a normal lifespan. The roadblock to this, again, is the cost—a curse that touches cancer patients everywhere. We must find a way to dispel that curse.

J. D. was only forty-six when he was diagnosed. Since we knew that his untimely death was preventable, it would have been wrenching for his family and me to accept such an ending. In the course of the days with my patients, when it seemed there was no light at the end of the tunnel for them or me, I remembered my voyage with J. D. and Sally.

PART 4

MRS. COOPER: THE OLDEST OLD AND CANCER

CHAPTER 15

Susan, a young RN in our hospital, came to talk to me. I had known her for three years.

"It's about my grandmother, Dr. Rahman," she said. "She's quite sick. They've found cancer cells in her abdominal fluid. She's eighty-seven years old. What should we do?"

"What does your grandmother want?" I asked.

"That's the problem—she's left it to me. I'm her only grandchild, and I mean the world to her. I may be wrong, but I'm afraid she'll agree to do things just to please me."

I promised to discuss the matter with her after I had seen her grandmother during my rounds.

Mrs. Cooper was thin and frail, with a swollen abdomen. Lying quietly in bed, eyes closed, she looked worn out. I could hear the faint hum of an IV pump as an intravenous fluid dripped into her left arm. I wondered if she would be able to give a good history. She opened her eyes as I gently tapped her shoulder. I introduced myself. A cancer doctor's visit means bad news, and I couldn't always be sure if my reception would be warm.

"I was expecting you," she said with a smile. "Susan thinks a lot of you. Thank you for coming to see me." Her outward appearance was deceptive. This woman was mentally sharp.

"How did your problem start, Mrs. Cooper?" I asked.

"I was married for sixty-eight years. My husband and I were farmers, and we also had some cattle. We worked together. Then Ed died of heart failure six months ago."

As usual, I was drawn to my patients' everyday lives, even though it took away more time from my practice. But Mrs. Cooper, like Corina Johnson, had a compelling way of beginning her story, so I let her go on.

"You can understand how hard it was for me," she said, tearing up. But she composed herself quickly. "A few months after his death, I began to lose my appetite. Since I wasn't that active anymore, I thought that was the reason. My family didn't agree. They said it was loneliness. I wasn't sure of that. I'd accepted his death. He'd been bedridden and miserable for fourteen months. Not being able to go to the fields or tend our stock was hard on him."

Her daughter, Molly, lived in a small town, and she had urged her mother to move in with her. But Mrs. Cooper refused.

"Ed and I had lived in the country our whole lives," she said. "We'd built our farm and homestead over the years. I couldn't abandon the place because he was gone. I still feel him in the house."

Molly gave in to her mother's wishes, and though she lived fifty miles away, she visited her mother as often as she could. In far West Texas, fifty miles isn't considered too long a distance.

Mrs. Cooper continued to lose weight and became weak. She went to her family physician. "The doctor gave me the same impression my children did," she said, "that I suffered from the unhappiness of a lonely widow."

After her husband's death, she managed her farm with hired hands.

"A farmer has to worry about weather, crops, and prices all the time," she added. "I thought if I got rid of those worries, I might improve. So I rented my land to a neighboring farmer. He thought a lot of my husband. Ed helped him when he was a young man and new to farming."

Then she added with a sad note, "None of my children is interested in having the farm. I don't blame them—they saw how hard we worked and still struggled. They have regular jobs in the towns. The younger generations are more interested in a stable income, and they don't care to live an isolated life."

Besides Molly, she had two sons. "The boys live in another state and are too busy with their own families," she said. "They visit me whenever they can."

But getting rid of the farm worries didn't help Mrs. Cooper's health.

"I developed stomachache and gas and bloating, and I had nausea. I went on a bland diet, hoping that would help. I gave up the Mexican food I loved."

Her abdominal gas and bloating increased, however, and she got short of breath while walking. Though eating less, she gained weight. She thought she had heart trouble like her husband's. He, too, had gained weight from fluid retention.

"I was reconciled that I would die like him," she said.

Then one day, she had sharp abdominal pain and vomiting. That was when she was brought to the hospital in San Angelo, more than a hundred miles from her farm. Her admitting diagnosis was "bowel obstruction."

A CT scan of the abdomen didn't show any blockage but showed ascites. Ascites is the accumulation of fluid between the two peritoneal linings, the tough membranes that encase the bowel. This fluid was the main culprit for her abdominal swelling. Ascites is always an ominous sign and is most commonly caused by advanced cirrhosis of the liver. But she rarely drank alcohol and had no history of hepatitis, the usual causes for cirrhosis.

Ascites, in reality, is peritoneal effusion, and its formation and management are similar to those of the pleural effusion, discussed in part 2 on Corina Johnson and her metastatic breast cancer.

Mrs. Cooper's abdominal fluid was pushing her diaphragm upwards and pressing on her lungs, resulting in shortness of breath, like the pleural fluid did. The admitting doctor did paracentesis: removal of fluid by puncturing the abdominal wall with a wide-bore needle, which was attached to a catheter that ran into a bag, where the fluid collected. This relieved the pressure on the diaphragm and eased her breathing. The drained fluid was sent for lab tests, as was done with the pleural fluid.

Paradoxically, even with all the water in her abdomen, she was still dehydrated from vomiting. The dehydration was due to a mechanism called "third-spacing," in which intravascular liquid moves out of the circulation and goes into another space—in her case, into the peritoneal cavity. Fluid is essential to the body's cells for metabolic activity, but they can't use the third-space liquid. For that reason, while the ascites is drained, patients also get IV hydration to correct the dehydration.

Her pathology report from the ascites noted "adenocarcinoma cells are present."

"My family is more shocked than I am," Mrs. Cooper said. "They feel bad for blaming things on loneliness. I'll accept whatever comes. This isn't my first bad news. Ed and I went through a lot."

Later, Susan and Molly and I came to her bedside.

"What do you recommend, Dr. R?" Susan asked. "I'm having difficulty explaining it all to my grandma, but she's understanding." Then she pointed to Molly and said, "My mom expects me to have all the answers just because I'm a nurse."

I sympathized with Susan. She was carrying the burden of being a medical professional, especially the only one in the family; in case of a medical dilemma, your loved ones turn to you for answers.

"I'm sorry, I can't recommend anything yet," I said.

"What do you mean?" Molly asked. "The report says cancer."

"Adenocarcinoma by itself is an incomplete diagnosis."

Then I went into detail about the nature of the problem. Adenocarcinoma originates from various organs in our body, such as the breast, colon, lung, pancreas, stomach, and ovary. So, the cancer could have come from any of them, but the response to treatments varies widely. For example, breast and ovarian cancers are treatable even in advanced stages, while pancreatic cancer is difficult to treat at any stage.

"Can't you tell from her CT scan of the abdomen where the cancer is from?" Molly asked.

"Her CT shows some vague changes in the ovaries and fluid in the abdomen. The fluid makes it hard for the radiologists to interpret the CT."

"What do we do now?"

"I've ordered a special blood test called cancer antigen 125 or CA 125. It's a tumor marker. Certain markers go up in certain cancers, and sometimes they help us to pinpoint a diagnosis."

At this point, Mrs. Cooper turned towards me. She smiled and said, "I hope I'm intelligent enough to take part in the discussion."

I immediately knew what I had done and apologized. I had made a common mistake. When very old patients come to see their doctors with their families, physicians tend to direct their attention to the latter, ignoring the patients, as if being elderly and frail made them incapable of comprehending anything. All this time, I had been looking at Susan and Molly and talking to them, without even glancing at the patient. I was humbled by Mrs. Cooper's subtlety in pointing out my error.

Her CA 125 result came back in two days—it was 3,600. CA 125 is a special protein secreted by cancer cells, but normal cells can also produce some. However, the normal level is less than thirty. The sky-high CA 125 in the presence of adenocarcinoma cells in the ascitic fluid clinched the diagnosis of ovarian cancer.

I explained all this to Mrs. Cooper. She took it better than Susan and Molly.

"I told you to see your gynecologist regularly," Susan admonished her grandmother. "Now you see what's happened."

"I saw my gynecologist two years ago," Mrs. Cooper said.

"That's not enough," Susan replied.

It was obvious that the young woman was afraid of losing her grandmother. Seeing where the discussion was heading, I intervened.

"It may not have made any difference how frequently she went for an exam," I said. "Ovarian cancer is notorious for staying hidden, and only about 15 percent of the tumors are detected at an early stage. Most ovarian cancers are advanced by the time they're diagnosed."

Mrs. Cooper gave me a look of appreciation for defending her. I realized she wanted to avoid any discord with her beloved granddaughter. Molly, too, wanted to change the subject.

"Where did the fluid come from if the cancer is in the ovary?" she asked.

"The cancer has spread to the lining of the bowel and caused the fluid."

"Can it come back like it did with my dad's heart trouble?"

"Yes, fluid from cancer always comes back unless the cancer is controlled."

"It seems the cancer is the source of all my troubles," Mrs. Cooper said.

"It is," I agreed.

"Can surgery take it all out?" Susan asked.

"Not in this case— it's advanced already."

"What do we do then?"

"Chemotherapy first to shrink the tumor, and then decide about surgery."

Susan was surprised about giving chemo before an operation.

"In my general surgery service, tumors are taken out first. Then the patients are sent for chemo if it's necessary."

"That's true in an early cancer, but when it's at a higher stage, chemo is often given first to reduce the tumor's size to make it operable."

From their expressions, I sensed that I had stirred a hornet's nest.

"At my age, Doctor, I'm not sure it's all worth it," Mrs. Cooper said.

"You've never given up on anything that I know of," countered Susan.

"That was a different time, Susan. I'm not young anymore."

Molly hadn't voiced her opinion so far, so I asked her, "What do you think?"

"I'll do whatever my mom wants."

"At least let's hear what kind of chemo Dr. R is talking about," Susan said. "I'm sure he's seen plenty of old people with cancer. Grandma isn't the only one."

There was palpable tension between Susan and the two older women. There's nothing easy about making life-and-death decisions, and it's not uncommon to see a generational gap in thinking among family members. It helps to give them time to sort things out.

Susan had brought up an important point about the elderly. Their numbers are increasing by leaps and bounds. The fastest growing population in the United States is the age group eighty-five years and older. They are now designated as "oldest old." Sooner or later, like Molly and Susan, almost every family in the nation will face similar dilemmas in handling their loved ones' critical years. Moreover, the incidence of cancer increases as we age. The oldest old represent 8 percent of all new cancer cases per year. In 2019, in this group alone, there were approximately 141,000 new cancer cases and 103,000 deaths.

San Angelo is a destination for many elderly retirees, so I had my share of oldest old patients. Practicing oncologists like me faced a systemic problem in medicine: there was hardly any practical information on chemotherapy for the oldest old. Clinical trials for cancer had so far excluded them. An attitude of "Why bother with cancer treatment if you are that old?" had permeated both medicine and society. When it came to chemo, advanced age and advanced cancer were often deemed mutually exclusive. Even taking into account all of the health difficulties the oldest old face—comorbidities, cognitive decline, and functional impairment—undertreatment of their cancer is still a factor.

The issue couldn't be easily dismissed. Being academic about someone's care is fine in abstract theory, but not so when you are at the bedside of an individual patient like Mrs. Cooper, especially when you know that effective chemo is available for her tumor—chemo that you wouldn't hesitate to give to younger patients who were equally ill or worse. In the past, having seen for years the disparity in caring for the elderly sick, in another context, I made an impassioned plea on their behalf in an article in the *New York Times* on January 23, 1986: "As a compassionate society, we must make a decision, here and now, whether we have a commitment to the elderly or whether we will abandon them when they need us most."

Having taken that stand, I was now caught in my own conflict. I knew that chronological age had less bearing on deciding chemotherapy; it was the functional status of the patients—how they manage their daily lives on their own—that mattered more. A forty-year-old person with bad cirrhosis and ascites and cancer would do worse than an active, otherwise healthy oldest old person with cancer. Mrs. Cooper's condition was obviously poor. Should I then send her to die in a hospice?

CHAPTER 16

My own uncertainty about making the decision on Mrs. Cooper worsened when the pathologist sent me an addendum report. He had done further cytology—study of cells—on her ascitic fluid and had found quite a few high-grade malignant cells. What did this mean? Tumors are categorized according to their rate of growth, defined as low, moderate, and high grade. A higher grade means faster growth and a poorer prognosis. In the past, almost all patients with high-grade ovarian cancer who were in Mrs. Cooper's condition died within a few months.

But that was no longer true. Two landmark drugs—Taxol and cisplatin (later, its less-toxic version, carboplatin), derived from the metal platinum—had brought success in ovarian cancer treatment. They had prolonged patient survival and improved the quality of life. But again, there wasn't much to read about their use in the eighty-five years old plus cohort. As always, I had to believe in myself before I could ask others to believe in me. There were times when I wasn't sure about what to do with some of the oldest old, and I had advised them to seek a second opinion. But many had refused this advice outright because they had decided against chemo to start with. I felt ashamed at how relieved I was by their decision, for they had rescued me from my own impasse.

After thinking things through, I concluded that Mrs. Cooper was a candidate for chemo, if she was willing to take it. For though she was quite sick at present, not too long before she had been physically active and running her own affairs. And she had been mentally sharp all along, sick or not. By now, I had seen enough old farming and ranching women from the countryside who had tolerated chemo better than women of the same age in New York or Houston.

I went back to Mrs. Cooper. Molly and Susan were there. I didn't know what had transpired between them, but Mrs. Cooper wanted to know her treatment options, including chemo. None of them was ready yet to accept hospice. At least for now, this made it easier for me. I brought up the chemo with Taxol and carboplatin. Upon hearing of Taxol, Susan, being a nurse, perked up.

"I was going to ask you about that," she said. "I've read about Taxol in the nursing magazines. They extract it from the bark of the Pacific yew tree. It's supposed to cure cancer. People were even stealing the bark to treat themselves."

What she was talking about was Taxol's intriguing history. When its clinical trials showed promise, it became the subject of the same hype that happens with the new anticancer drugs. But the premature limelight on Taxol had a unique and unfortunate effect: it devastated the Pacific yew. The natural history of this small-to medium-sized evergreen tree didn't serve it well. The active ingredient of its bark that destroys the cancer is paclitaxel. But to produce it in therapeutic doses, a large amount of bark is necessary. Harvesting the bark kills the trees. Since the drug was not yet ready for FDA approval, poachers stripped the bark from the yews, mixed it with legitimate sources, and sold it to licensed companies. Some even gathered it in the hopes of treating their own cancers, even though it was a futile exercise. Extracting paclitaxel from the bark is a complex procedure, and the bootleggers never got an effective dose. Both the yews and the patients suffered. Yews grow slowly, and some that had taken up to 200 years to grow were denuded in minutes. In a few places, the trees virtually disappeared. Environmentalists raised the alarm, though they garnered little sympathy from some corners. One of my own patients asked me bluntly, "If you had a choice, would you save me or save the yew?"

Fortunately, paclitaxel, in the brand name of Taxol, was soon manufactured as a semisynthetic compound and was made commercially available after FDA clearance. As time went on, it was found to be of broad benefit not only for ovarian cancer but also for cancer of the breast and other malignancies. To date, it's one of the best plant-based anticancer drugs besides vincristine.

Giving Taxol and carboplatin (carbo) simultaneously had a higher response rate than giving either of them alone. The combination, therefore, was the standard for ovarian cancer. But once more, I couldn't go by the book, because two drugs would have more complications than one, and we were in an uncharted territory. Would an eighty-seven-year-old body be able to bear the toxicities, regardless of what Mrs. Cooper's constitution had been before? I had some doubts. If I treated her, I would try the easier of the two: carbo.

Though Susan was a dedicated surgical nurse, she had stayed away from the cancer unit and chemotherapy in particular. She couldn't escape the uneasiness that some doctors and nurses felt about chemo, fearing it was too complex, even when it was not. But now, with her grandmother's diagnosis, chemo came close to home.

"Do you want to try Taxol for Grandma, Dr. R?" she asked.

"I'm not sure if it's right for her because of its toxicity."

I discussed myelosuppression and its consequences, like infection and bleeding. Then Taxol's propensity for causing bone and joint pain, in addition to peripheral neuropathy, especially in Mrs. Cooper's age group.

"The Taxol articles don't say much about these things," Susan said. "I shouldn't have brought it up in front of Grandma."

"I'm glad you did," Mrs. Cooper said. "He proves my point. It's not worth going through all those troubles at my age."

Had I made my own mistake by mentioning Taxol? Giving the whole picture was the right thing to do. But, was it necessary to give the whole picture all at once and turn off the patient? First, I should have emphasized carbo, which was my choice to begin with.

Susan countered her grandmother's reluctance. "Dr. R hasn't discussed carboplatin yet, Grandma."

"Of course," I said, looking at Mrs. Cooper, "carboplatin is easier to tolerate. And compared to Taxol, it's also easier to give through an IV."

"I'm not sure I understand what you mean by something made from platinum," Mrs. Cooper said.

I was pleased by her curiosity. I briefly told her the history of carboplatin and how it was derived from cisplatin, the first metal-based anticancer drug.

"It's interesting, how medicines are discovered," she said.

"So you don't have any reservations about it?" Susan asked me.

"It has one particular side effect that I worry about. Though other blood counts don't go down much, platelets can drop a lot, and that can cause bruises and bleeding. But we can watch the blood counts closely."

"Then let's just forget about the treatment. I've lived long enough," Mrs. Cooper said.

Susan wasn't about to give up. "I want to have you around longer, Grandma," she said. "Give it at least one try. If it makes you too sick, I'll be the first one to stop it."

Then she said something in earnest, as if to convince me. "Grandma has always been thin, and she walks with slow steps. People who don't know her mistake her for a frail woman, especially when she's sick. But she's tough as nails. She wasn't just a farmer's wife—she was a farmer herself. Grandpa said he wouldn't have made it without her."

Molly had been watching her mother and daughter debate it out. I sensed that she felt caught between them and wasn't sure what course to take, except that she was likely to support her mother. But now she seemed to take her daughter's side: "Susan is right about Mom's toughness."

Although Susan wanted Mrs. Cooper to have the treatment, I was obligated to honor the patient's wishes, not the granddaughter's, even if I understood the latter's sentiment. Therefore, after discussing the pros and cons of carbo, I asked Mrs. Cooper plainly, "Do you really want the chemo?"

"I should give it a try for her," she said, smiling at Susan. The young nurse gave a sigh of relief. I reflexively looked at Molly. "I'll do what Mom wants," she said again.

After infusion, carbo is cleared by the kidneys, so its dose is calculated according to the level of kidney function—that is, the lower the function, the lower the dose. Like with other organs and tissues, the strength of the kidneys and bone marrow decline as we age; that's the way the body's physiological processes work. There was not much solid information on the state of the kidneys of Mrs. Cooper's demographic, so I had to be extra careful in deciding the dose.

We cautiously gave her the first chemo. Except for fatigue and mild nausea, she managed it well, which eased our tension.

She was sent home and was to return in three weeks for the next treatment. While Susan checked on her regularly, I did the same with her CBC. To be sure, her blood counts dropped, but they stayed within a safe range.

In three weeks, she looked stronger and was eating and drinking better. She had some residual ascites after it was drained in the hospital, but that, too, had diminished. This meant she had a responsive tumor. Mrs. Cooper herself was surprised by her changes. Besides, with all the bad things I had said to her about the chemo, nothing serious had happened.

Encouraged, she received the second cycle of carbo, and her ascites almost completely cleared up. She drove to her farm in the mornings to watch things. Going to the fields always made her happy. As with everything else, improvement begets improvement, and she was more active. That made us comfortable in administering the third treatment.

Susan came to my office with a bouquet of flowers for my nurses and other staff. By now, Mrs. Cooper had become the grandmother of everyone—nurses, office assistants, and lab techs. They looked forward to her heartwarming smile, a smile that stayed put despite what we were doing to her. And she, too, loved them all.

"I can't thank you enough," Susan said to me.

"You deserve the credit. She went for chemo because of you. You were right about her being hardy."

"You wouldn't believe how much my little boy adores her and how much she enjoys his company. I used to be scared of letting them spend time together, because I was worried about transmitting infection. Not anymore. My mother laughs at their antics. One three-year-old and another eighty-seven. She says I have two children now. My boy is lucky. How many kids have a chance to see four generations together?"

After the fourth cycle of carbo, Mrs. Cooper's CA 125 came down close to normal. A repeat abdominal CT also brought good news: the ascites was gone, and the ovarian changes that we saw in the CT before the chemo had resolved.

To reiterate: if ovarian cancer is diagnosed early, it's first treated with surgery by removing all the female organs—the uterus, ovaries, and fallopian tubes. But with an inoperable cancer, the order of the treatment is reversed, with chemo first to shrink the tumor to an operable size.

We had surely reduced Mrs. Cooper's tumor, with visible improvement of her symptoms. Could we now adhere to the rules and do the surgery? Not necessarily. She wasn't a younger woman, and surgery and anesthesia had risks. At eighty-seven, how long could we prolong her life safely?

Yet, we couldn't ignore some unique aspects of ovarian cancer. It's notorious for seeding the peritoneal surfaces of the abdomen and pelvis with tiny tumors known as implants—the reason for ascites. Unfortunately, many of these implants are too small to be visible on CT. So even a normal-looking

CT isn't a guarantee that all the tumors are gone. Left alone, these implants would grow and cause many complications that I worried about. One was the formation of extensive scars, which would strangle and obstruct the bowel, at times so complex that they couldn't be released by surgery. If Mrs. Cooper developed these problems, all the progress she had made so far would come to nothing. Therefore, post-chemo resection of any possible remaining tumor was important to obtain CR and prevent recurrence.

I again debated the persistent issue: should I decide on the basis of her age alone or the quality of her present life? As with chemotherapy, I had to be sure myself before I brought it to her.

I thought about one of my heroes in medicine, Dr. Michael E. DeBakey. He was a giant in cardiovascular surgery and the undisputed leader at Baylor College of Medicine in Houston, where I had much of my US training. His patients, kings to commoners, came from all over the world, and many of his cases were too risky to be operated on by other surgeons. Among other medical residents and fellows at BCM, I had to see some of his patients for pre-op consultation with the help of our attendings and professors. Even though we feared DeBakey and avoided him if we could, owing to his stern manner, we admired him for his skill and medical leadership. Among his many achievements, he was the pioneer in repairing abdominal aortic aneurysm (AAA), caused by thinning and ballooning of the aorta, the biggest artery in the body. Rupture of an AAA is fatal unless it's operated on promptly.

As his luck would have it, once, DeBakey's own aorta was about to rupture, which put him into a coma and almost killed him. He was ninety-seven. There was intense debate among the renowned BCM doctors whether to let him die or try to save him. The first group surmised that he couldn't survive the anesthesia and the perilous operation at his age, and in his dire state, it would be unethical to submit him to surgery. But the second group thought he should be given a chance. And surprisingly, for a person of his stature, Dr. DeBakey had left confusing medical directives for himself. His family, however, backed surgery. After some debate, he underwent the very operation that he had pioneered. Who performed this hazardous task? It was none other than his protégé, George Noon. (Noon was a junior faculty member at BCM when I was there, and was well-liked, especially by the trainees, because of his amiable manner and his commitment to patients. He has stayed at BCM and made huge contributions to cardiovascular surgery.)

After a rocky post-op course, DeBakey recovered well, living about two more productive years. Being oldest old was not a dead end. This case is also a glaring example of medical ethics at the bedside, as opposed to propounding it as a theoretical academic exercise.

Of course, Mrs. Cooper wasn't Dr. DeBakey, and she had neither his privilege nor his disease. Yet, she was ten years younger and was certainly in better shape than he was. More important, she was not in a coma and was mentally competent to make her own decisions. She, too, was a hero to me from what I had learned of her, though I realized being a hero wasn't a surgical criterion by itself. Even if I discarded my bias, I couldn't discard the fact that she had a treatable tumor and had responded well to chemo. Didn't she then deserve all the chances we could offer? It would be up to her to accept or reject them.

Her acceptance alone, however, wouldn't be enough to do the operation, and, as in many surgeries, we still had two more hurdles to clear. We had to decide if her heart, especially at her age and with her current medical problems, could endure the anesthesia and surgery. In addition, we had to determine if the surgery was technically feasible.

The cardiologist I consulted was surprised by the strength of her cardiac function and cleared her for surgery. Then I sent her to Dr. H, an accomplished gynecologic surgeon. I tactfully avoided the gynecologist who had examined Mrs. Cooper during her original admission. From the start, his attitude had been like that of some of the doctors who see cancer in her age group and say, "What's the use?" In contrast, Dr. H was sympathetic to these patients, and I appreciated her clinical approach. Besides, I trusted her because she, too, had the hallmark of a fine surgeon: good judgment and skill. She was impressed by how Mrs. Cooper had fought so far and how she had changed her life for the better. Dr. H carefully reviewed her records and thoroughly examined her, and decided that resection was feasible and appropriate, but with moderate risk.

Dr. H discussed the surgery and its benefits and risks with Mrs. Cooper and her family, and they all felt comfortable with her. Even so, I wanted to reassure myself, so I got together with them again.

"What do you think, Molly?" I asked her first since she usually seemed to stay back.

Her answer was predictable. "Whatever Mom decides is all right with me."

Before I could ask Mrs. Cooper, Susan looked at her and said, "You should have the operation, Grandma. See how much better you are now?" Then she made a comment to fortify her assertion, "I have faith in Dr. R."

Mrs. Cooper softly laughed and said, "Susan puts too much burden on you, Dr. Rahman. I hope you understand her." Then she added, "Go ahead with the operation."

We waited a few weeks until her CBC was good enough and she had done more physical activity. After that, the resection was performed. My trust in Dr. H's dexterous hands was validated. There were no unusual incidents during the surgery. We observed Mrs. Cooper closely and kept our fingers crossed. Sometimes the good of an operation is negated by the bad of the post-op complications.

We anxiously awaited the all-important pathology report on the surgical specimens. What would the pathologist find? A lot of cancer still? Or a little of it or none? Was this all worth it for Mrs. Cooper? It was the one report that would give us the answers and the make-or-break verdict.

CHAPTER 17

T he pathology report confirmed that Mrs. Cooper's cancer had indeed originated in the ovaries. "Necrotic tumor in the left ovary, with viable malignant cells present," the pathologist noted. In plain English, this meant that the carboplatin (carbo) had killed most of the cancer cells but not all.

Dr. H's surgical findings were also revealing. The patient's peritoneal surfaces in the abdomen and pelvis were studded with the characteristic ovarian cancer implants. The smaller ones had completely necrosed—died—while the larger ones still had residual cancer. The lymph nodes that were removed as a part of the surgery to determine the extent of the tumor showed similar results: a few living cells among the dead ones. Hence, Mrs. Cooper indeed had an advanced disease, at least stage three out of the maximum four.

Although the pathology report made it sound like the chemo had been a failure, it was, in fact, a success—she got a partial remission. This is the way ovarian cancer—for that matter, all cancers—behave on the way to possible CR. Unlike with the visible implants, neither the x-rays and scans nor the naked eye can see microscopic disease left behind. In time, this microscopic cancer, like the visible implants, raises its ugly head and leads to progression or recurrence.

Thankfully, Mrs. Cooper didn't have any major post-op setbacks. The potential complications we had feared didn't happen. She couldn't, however, escape our iatrogenic effect: urinary tract infection from the urinary catheter, which she needed during the anesthesia and until she was able to void on her own in a few days. Unlike Clara Anderson's infection detailed in part 1, this was an uncomplicated infection, and it was easily cleared with an antibiotic.

A few weeks after the surgery, Susan came to see me again by herself. She was concerned about the pathology report—the persistence of cancer—though I had amply warned her, her grandmother, and her mother ahead of time that this could be a likely outcome.

"Still, I was hoping it was all gone," Susan said, "the way Grandma bounced back and regained her energy after the chemo."

"Tumor load and how you function are inversely related," I explained. "The less cancer you have, the better your energy. That's what happened to your grandma—when the chemo reduced the tumor volume, she felt better."

"What can we do for the remaining cancer?"

I had to tell her about cancer's biological facts. Since carbo had shrunk Mrs. Cooper's cancer, chemo could still work, especially since her tumor size was smaller now. But any advanced cancer like Mrs. Cooper's was duplicitous, and the chances of chemo resistance were higher with a single drug than with combination chemo.

"Then do you want to add Taxol? She's stronger now."

"I've been thinking of that. The two together may put her into complete remission, but it's hard to say for how long."

"I know you'll do the right thing."

"We need to get together again to talk about treatment."

We did. I explained to Mrs. Cooper and Molly what I had explained to Susan.

"Susan and you have been right so far," Mrs. Cooper said. "I'll keep my part of the bargain. Go ahead with your plan."

I was expecting that she would have some reservations. Either Susan had convinced her well, or she was ready on her own, seeing how the chemo had made a difference.

I gave her the first cycle of the Taxol and carbo combination. It wasn't a surprise that she had more myelosuppression, but it didn't fall into the risky range. At the next follow-up, I questioned her closely.

"To tell you the truth," she said, "the aches and pains are bothersome, but I can handle it. Ibuprofen helps. But the tingling and numbness in my hands and feet are hard to take. I didn't have those before."

I did a neurological examination and found her to have peripheral neuropathy. No matter how much I had tried *not* to make decisions based solely on her age, I had to admit this: it was her age that made her more prone to nerve damage from Taxol. However, this degree of neurological symptoms coming on so quickly didn't make sense.

I tried to remember if I had run into this kind of situation before, and my mind clicked on another elderly woman whose symptoms had been like Mrs. Cooper's: tingling, numbness, and aches and pains in the extremities. She saw various doctors and underwent all sorts of tests, including invasive angiograms to rule out circulatory problems, but no cause was found. Thinking of any possible obscure cancer, she was referred to me. But she had no cancer—all she had was peripheral neuropathy from a vitamin B12 deficiency. The lack of vitamin B12 is notorious for causing damage to the nervous system. However, she had an extremely unusual form of B12 problem, so it was easy to miss. By sheer luck and a high index of suspicion, I was able to identify the issue. The woman was easily treated with simple, inexpensive B12 injections—first often and then monthly. In time, her symptoms resolved. She taught me so much that I presented a paper on her at a medical conference in New York City.

Could Mrs. Cooper then also have a B12 deficiency on top of her chemotherapy burden? An uncomplicated test—checking the B12 level in the blood—found it out. Sure enough, it was quite low, which must have added to her Taxol side effects. Her neurological symptoms, too, subsided with the B12 treatment.

Mrs. Cooper's case is one more reminder that other concomitant diseases can exacerbate chemo toxicities, which can be mistakenly attributed to the chemo alone. Oncologists encounter these sorts of pitfalls more often than other physicians. Chemo patients also carry an unfortunate mark, as if a scarlet letter, justified or not. Sometimes all their past and current troubles are unjustly blamed on their cancer and chemo. But even outside cancer, it's not uncommon for doctors to say to the elderly when they come with complaints: "It's just from old age."

With the amelioration of Mrs. Cooper's neuropathy, we came to another turn on our path: to decide whether to give the second cycle of the combination chemo. We couldn't wait too long, for it was a tug-of-war between looming death from the tumor progression versus being disabled by the increasing nerve damage. Ultimately, I concluded that, having made major gains, it wouldn't be right to abandon the treatment, and if she was willing to take a chance, I would be willing, too.

I had a heart-to-heart talk with Mrs. Cooper. "I can't guarantee that the neuropathy won't get worse if we repeat the chemo, but I also worry that your cancer will grow back if we don't."

She thought for a while, then said, "You've been complaining about not having enough information and knowledge on an eighty-seven-year-old. Maybe your experience with my cancer will help you to help others like me. I've lived long enough to know that nothing is guaranteed in life. But I've made it so far because of the chemo, so I'll continue."

What she said about gaining knowledge about the oldest old had been in the back of my mind, but I couldn't quite articulate it myself due to my personal doubts. Once again, it was a patient who rescued me from my own impasse, while at the same time teaching me about altruism.

Susan, of course, was for staying with the plan, which was to give a total of three cycles of the combination and then recheck the tumor status. We went ahead and administered the second chemo.

While waiting three to four weeks for her to be ready for the third, I got a call from the ER. Ominously again, it came in the middle of the night.

"Mrs. Cooper is here," the ER doctor said. "She was brought in by an ambulance. She has epistaxis [nosebleed]. I've packed her nose, but the packing is quickly getting soaked with blood. Her platelets have dropped to only 9,000. I've ordered platelet transfusion."

I immediately got up and got dressed to go to the ER. Ara was used to this kind of intrusion, and she bore it with patience. Seeing me still a bit groggy, she said, "Drink a cup of hot tea before you leave, and pay attention to your driving."[3]

Once I reached the ER and saw Mrs. Cooper, I realized I had been told only half the story. She looked as if she had been mauled by an animal. Bright red blood from her nose had soaked her blouse despite the nasal packing. She had extensive bruises on her arms, chest, back, and face. With just 9,000 platelets (normal is 150,000 to 450,000), her blood was clotting very poorly. I was, of course, concerned about her external bleeding, but it was the fear

---

3 In the mid-1970s, when I began my practice in San Angelo as a young doctor, a few times my wife and I were awakened at night by loud knocks at our door, and a policeman would be standing there with a message from the hospital. This happened because sometimes we were so deeply asleep holding each other that we missed the ringing of our telephone. The first time the police came, I was bewildered and scared until the officer told me the reason for his coming. In those days, we managed well despite having only basic means of communication.

of internal hemorrhage that panicked me most—bleeding into the brain or the abdominal organs would be fatal to her. She would need many platelet transfusions to prevent this calamity.

As sometimes happens in any hospital, that night, we were short of platelets. A trauma surgeon needed them for emergency surgeries, and an eighty-seven-and-a-half-year-old with cancer wasn't a priority for the blood bank.

"Mrs. Cooper's cancer is in remission," I said to the blood bank supervisor to persuade her, even though I knew that, so far, only her cancer marker, CA125, had returned to normal, and we were yet to document a CR. "You can't let her die now because of hemorrhage. What would you do if she were your grandmother?"

The supervisor got me bags of platelets from another hospital, and they were quickly infused. Soon, Mrs. Cooper's nosebleed stopped. She also had significant anemia from blood loss and received multiple blood transfusions.

Thrombocytopenia—a low platelet count—is a dose-limiting factor for carboplatin and as with other chemo, it's cumulative. For that reason, we had kept a close watch on Mrs. Cooper's platelet levels, and whenever they had dropped, they had rebounded in time. The last chemo, however, must have broken the threshold that the platelets could withstand.

The sad part of chemo is that it's still primitive, no matter how we claim otherwise. The aim is to destroy only cancer cells, but the collateral damage is unavoidable, for the drugs don't discriminate between the good and the bad cells. Hence, even with all the precautions, one can't avoid the unpredictable: things can be going along smoothly, then suddenly they are *not*.

Susan had the hardest time seeing her grandmother this way, and her sobbing was ceaseless.

"Why did I push her to take the chemo?" she kept saying. "Why did I ask for Taxol? She was doing well with the carbo alone."

It was hard enough to witness Mrs. Cooper's suffering and her frightening nosebleed and bruises, and now here was this young woman's heartbreaking anguish. I fought not to break down in front of her.

"Don't blame yourself," I consoled Susan. "I'm her oncologist, and I'm the one who gave her the chemo, not you." Then, to soothe her further, I emphasized, "Your grandma is a very intelligent woman, and she'd have refused the chemo if she didn't want it. We can't undo what's been done. You must pull yourself together for her sake."

Mrs. Cooper remained stable with the transfusions. At her bedside, I grappled for something profound to say, but the only words that came to me were: "I'm sorry for putting you through this."

She tried to put me at ease. "Things happen in life," she said. "You didn't want this just as I didn't."

I wished she would question my judgment or show some anger toward me. But she realized how badly Susan was taking things, and how I, too, was having a hard time of it. Molly had her mother's stoicism, and that helped a lot.

In about ten days or so, her platelets began to come up, then they climbed quickly once the bone marrow had recovered. Her bruises faded away slowly, and her WBC and hemoglobin rose. She was ready to go home.

Throughout Mrs. Cooper's hospitalization, Molly had given me quiet and consistent support, but had stayed unobtrusive. During the discharge, however, she pulled me aside and said, "Thank you, Dr. Rahman, for being there for both my mother and daughter."

It's mostly the daughters who take care of the elderly parents. But whether daughters or sons, many of these children are, by then, elderly themselves. Molly was going to take her mother to her home, and she herself was sixty-seven years old. As the baby boom generation gets progressively older, their care will become increasingly harder.

After a few weeks with Molly, Mrs. Cooper got restless. "I don't like town," she said. It was a town of only one thousand people, but that was still too much for her. Her newfound strength reinforced her desire to return to her own home.

"I want to be in my farmhouse and fields," she said to me. "Susan is asking me to live with her in San Angelo. But it's a big city, I feel lost there. I come to San Angelo because of my doctors."

"San Angelo is a small city," I countered.

She laughed. "You've lived in New York City and Houston, so nothing looks big to you." She also brought up a matter that was bothering her.

"If I can help it, I don't want to be a burden to my daughter and granddaughter. They have good hearts, and they've been good to me. How many ill mothers and grandmothers can say that these days? But they're busy with their own lives, and I don't want to impose on them."

Patients and their families share their doubts and problems with the doctors they trust. Inevitably, one sometimes finds oneself caught between the conflicting sides. If you take one side, the other side gets unhappy. But being on the patients' side may not be enough either, because they have their limitations. Still, I was for granting Mrs. Cooper's wish.

"If going back to your place means that much to you, do you want me talk to Molly and Susan?" I asked her.

"That'll help. If you okay it, they won't fuss."

"I'll try."

Since she'd been discharged from the hospital, neither of us had brought up her cancer or chemo. I felt she had had enough of the treatment, and now what would happen would happen.

Although Molly didn't favor her mother living by herself, she might relent to my advice, but I was unsure of Susan. She was forceful and protective when it came to her grandmother. I approached each woman separately.

"Your mom is active now and not on chemo," I said to Molly. "I share your concern, but you should let her have her wish."

"I knew sooner or later she was going to ask you to do this. I'm willing to let her try, but you better explain it to Susan first."

I called Susan to drop by my office.

"I'm not asking you to give any more chemo to Grandma," she said when she came in.

"It's not that, I'm stopping the treatment."

"What then?"

"She wants to return to her farm."

"It's all right with me if that makes her happy."

It took me a few seconds to take in her answer. That she didn't argue at all astonished me.

"Have you given any thought to it before?" I asked.

"Yes. Since she got well, I knew this was coming. She loves her place as if my grandpa is still living there."

"I am sure she'll appreciate your understanding."

"When we almost lost her, I thought about things I had avoided before. And I realized I was acting to protect my own feelings, not my grandmother's."

It's amazing how well patients can do when the weight of the chemo is out of the way. Besides, Mrs. Cooper's surroundings and the country air did something to her. She seemed rejuvenated, even as she neared eighty-eight.

Though she was no longer on treatment, we enjoyed seeing each other off and on. I didn't do any more scans or x-rays. The only thing I asked for was the marker CA 125, which had dropped to normal since her last chemo, fateful as it was. The test was more to satisfy my need than for her benefit; we both knew if the marker went up again, we wouldn't intervene with chemo. To assuage my guilt for continuing the CA 125, she reminded me what she had said in the past about helping others. "There're plenty of old folks with cancer. The test will find out how long this chemo will keep working. That should give you a clue for how to take care of them."

This was one benevolent soul, and I felt lucky to be a part of her life. As the months passed, our friendship deepened.

CHAPTER 18

I n some years, when it rains in time, Texas turns into a riot of colors in the spring, painted by wildflowers from Orange in East Texas to El Paso in far West Texas, a distance close to one thousand miles. Even the lifeless grounds of the desert bloom with such intensity that one would think there had never been a desert there. Ara and I have a passion for these untamed blooms, and on the weekends or holidays, when I could take off from work, we would take turns driving hundreds of miles to feast our eyes on them. This refreshed us more than anything else and quieted my restless mind. In my work, good news and bad news often came in cycles, but on occasion, the latter seemed relentless, with all its specter of death and dying. Ara knew that nature soothed me, even more so in her company. So, she encouraged me to take these wildflower adventure trips. She had been my constant support in my travails and trials, yet I had given her less time than she deserved. For at times, I was too preoccupied with the problems of my patients. Hence, these explorations were also my way of giving back to her a little.

Searching for the wildflowers year after year, we had come to know some remote corners of the countryside—in particular, the Hill Country of Texas, where the roadsides, fields, and ranches turn into magical carpets of blue-bonnets, the state flower. One lovely spring, Mrs. Cooper told me about her meadows: "Their beauty is unreal this year."

When I mentioned how much Ara and I loved wildflowers, she was delighted. "Why don't you two come to my place?"

The following weekend, we paid her a visit. Many country roads look alike, so even with the directions she gave me, it wasn't easy to find her place. West Texas is sparsely populated, and homesteads are few and far between. And her house stood on a bend of a narrow path. As we searched for her property, we stopped by a barn and saw an old man with a Stetson, blue jeans, and a faded shirt. His sunburnt face had a friendly countenance. He looked at us curiously as we stopped. After all, he wasn't used to seeing "foreign looking" persons driving around there, and one being a young lady in a sari at that. We asked him about Mrs. Cooper's house.

"A good woman," he said. "She's my neighbor." He told us how to find her farm. But his definition of "neighbor" was different from ours—Mrs. Cooper lived about twenty miles away.

When we arrived, Mrs. Cooper took Ara in her arms as if she were her granddaughter, and her face beamed. "I'm glad you've come to see me, Mrs. Rahman. Dr. Rahman has told me a lot about you. How lovely you are!" Ara was a beautiful woman all right, and she looked especially attractive in her colorful saris, glistening black hair down to her waist, and penetrating brown eyes in a handsome face. She was then in her early thirties.

"Thank you. You can call me Ara. My husband thinks a lot of you, Mrs. Cooper."

I had foreseen these conversations, so I had gotten Mrs. Cooper's permission ahead of time to tell of her diagnosis to Ara. The two women hit it off quickly.

Her dwelling was an old, three-bedroom house, unpretentious, with old furniture. But her window curtains and bedcovers were something else. They were immediately noticeable because of their intricate designs.

"These are beautiful!" Ara exclaimed.

"A few of them came from my mother a long time ago, but most of them I've embroidered myself over the years. The Lord has kept my eyesight good."

"Do you follow pictures or sketches for the designs?"

"I copy from nature—from the flowers, leaves, birds, and butterflies. I don't have any blueprint."

"You're a good artist."

"Thank you, Ara. I don't deserve the credit; all I do is to borrow from what I see in my surroundings. I'm not original."

She served pecan pie she had made for us. Then she gave us tea. I came to know that she didn't drink tea but drank coffee once in a while; she, too, had found out from my assistants that I loved hot tea. I ate the pie with relish, and after I finished, I mopped up the crumbs with my fingertips. She saw what I was doing.

"Have another piece," she said and put a big slice on my plate. I felt embarrassed.

"It's so delicious. You know the artistry of pie making."

"I've had long years of practice. It was Ed's favorite. I'm glad you like it."

Her house was on high ground. We sat on the porch and drank tea as we gazed at the landscape. There were splashes of color all around. Thick growths of bluebonnets stretched as far as the eye could see. From a distance, it looked as though the fields were a waving blue ocean, and we were sitting on an island. Mrs. Cooper reminded us of something that Texans of all stripes appreciate. "I'm glad Lady Bird Johnson did so much to encourage the cultivation and promotion of wildflowers. If nothing else, she got the attention of city folks like you." Then she smiled at Ara and said, "I hope you don't mind my saying this. It's good for you and your husband to refresh your minds. He has a hard enough job, and that can't be easy on you either."

Ara was touched and said, "You are so kind to think about us."

On one side of the house was a pond, and some wild ducks were frolicking and making a ruckus. I felt nostalgic. Memories flooded my mind about my past in Bangladesh—how our ponds, lakes, and marshes were home to all kinds of wild ducks and other birds. Our own family lake, named Patla Pukur—the pond of the light water—had an abundance of them. The lake was so named because a legend told us that, when weighed, its water was the lightest of all the waters. And it had healing powers. My grandmother dispensed it to us if we had any gastrointestinal ailments when I was growing up. Even after decades of being a high-tech doctor, I hadn't forgotten her remedy and how much I loved it.

Mrs. Cooper became animated. "You can see why I don't want to abandon this place."

I knew what she was getting at, and inadvertently, my doctor's side took over. "I'm sure Molly and Susan understand it, but they can't help worrying about your living alone. With all that you've been through with . . ."

Ara, sitting next to her, gave me a sharp look. I was there as a friend, not as an oncologist. There was no reason to bring up her cancer now, especially since she hadn't brought it up herself. We were having a pleasant time, and Ara didn't want me to spoil it.

Mrs. Cooper wanted to show us some old family pictures, and she took us into a side room, her small library. The room had a table and a chair, and a shelf with about two dozen books. From the titles on their spines, they were Bibles, inspirational books, and Westerns, including one classic, *The Time It Never Rained* by Elmer Kelton, one of the greatest Western writers of all time. I hadn't read many Western novels, but this was one book about West Texas that I admired a great deal. It vividly portrays a prolonged drought in the early 1950s in this part of the state, and its aftermath, with lives ruined and remade. As Kelton put it, "[It] was inspired by actual events, when the longest and the most severe drought in living memory pressed ranchers and farmers to the outer limits of their courage and endurance." The book resonated with me because I, myself, had taken care of some of those farmers and ranchers in their old years, and had heard their firsthand accounts.

I took the volume off the shelf and began to flip through it. "Kelton really knows farmers and ranchers as they are," Mrs. Cooper said. "That's because he lives among us."

"I know him well," I said. "He's lived in San Angelo most of his life. Besides being a top writer of Westerns, he's one of the finest human beings I know."

"That he is. I'm glad your paths have crossed."

"He is kind to me and encourages my writing."

"I'm so glad he did. You write very well."

There was a pile of newspapers on the table. While she was looking for the family pictures, I picked up an issue, and to my surprise, I saw her bylines on the front page.

"You're a reporter and a writer!" I exclaimed.

"Well, I've been reporting for fifty years. I try to share the stories of my far scattered neighbors."

"May I read them?"

"Sure."

Being careful about protecting my patients' privacy, I was struck by how personal her reportage was—news that, in my view, didn't belong in the public sphere. She noticed my astonished look when I saw my name in one of the issues, written in the third person. "Ivy Cooper saw her cancer specialist, Dr. Fazlur Rahman, a week ago. She got a good report on her cancer of the ovary. She appreciates her caring doctor."

"Well," she said, "in the isolated parts where we live, we like to know how things are going with our neighbors. It may look nosey to the city folks, but here we try to help each other in times of need. So knowing helps. The news also lists the names of the sick, and we pray for them in our churches, and raise money to help them with their medical bills. Besides, farming has a set routine, and sick or well, the planting and harvesting don't wait for us. We all pitch in when someone is unable to work."

She was a reporter for this biweekly sheet, published from a nearby small town, where her daughter lived. Ara asked her how she collected the news.

"Sometimes my friends call me with the information and sometimes I call them. I also visit people whenever I can. The families know me, and they like to share their stories. My regret is that I've missed a lot because of my cancer."

There was no big political news or anything earth-shattering in her paper. And no embellishments in her descriptions. Just plain, straightforward language—reporting births, deaths, weddings, illnesses, and other events in the life of ordinary people.

I couldn't help inquiring about her philosophy of journalism. She was surprised by my question.

"I don't have any big philosophy or unique method," she said. "I just observe and listen and then write it as it is. It works for me. I write with pen and paper, and a messenger comes to pick them up for printing."

Then she paused and said, "It's not writing like you do. I've read some of your articles reprinted in the *San Angelo Standard-Times*. Susan gave them to me. They're really good, and I've learned quite a few things from them. But I don't write on issues, I just relate what happens in our everyday lives."

Since I had first seen her in the hospital, I had often wondered how she could be so articulate, with such a good vocabulary. I knew she had had only limited schooling, and didn't she live far away from civilization and culture?

Now I realized it was my own hubris that had raised these questions, hubris I had picked up in my years in New York and Houston. Mrs. Cooper was such a humble soul that she had never mentioned her creative side. I wished I had her wisdom and her brevity in writing.

Before we left Mrs. Cooper, she asked us to take a turn out to a big pasture. "It's a fine place to see colors," she said. "You shouldn't miss it."

We followed her directions and found the field. We couldn't believe our eyes—from what we saw, it was as if we had landed on another planet. The bluebonnets by themselves were pretty enough, but Ara and I preferred other flowers mixed among them. And mixed they were: Indian paintbrush, Indian blanket, white and yellow daisies, black-eyed Susan, coreopsis, white poppies, verbenas, Mexican hats, Queen Anne's lace, grass flowers, and others whose names we didn't know. Nature's unseen hands had created a mystical bouquet.

Many of these flowers bloom at different intervals depending on the timing of the rains, but in some years, nature becomes more generous than usual and brings them out simultaneously. This Texas lushness is sometimes so impressive that magazines and newspapers from here and abroad gush about it.

Lest we forget this wasn't a garden but a pasture, cattle and horses were grazing around, and some of the cows were drinking and wallowing in a waterhole. Farmhouses and barns could be seen in the distance, along with a few oak groves. A running stream gurgled nearby. Streams in West Texas go dry without notice, so seeing and hearing this one made us happy, especially in this enchanted setting.

Ara and I felt like walking among the extravagant growth, but we remembered Mrs. Cooper's caution. "It's tempting to walk in the flowers," she warned, "but don't. Rattlesnakes lie hidden in the brush."

Beauty has its dangers. I dreaded rattlesnakes. They are ubiquitous in West Texas, and over the years, I had seen quite a few patients bitten by them. Among other things, a severe bite with high envenomation can induce critical blood-clotting problems, resulting in horrible hemorrhage from all the pores in the body. You can never forget some of these patients. But the truth is that snakes try to avoid humans and inflict harm only when they are disturbed or surprised.

Ara and I scanned the countryside in all directions. The sun was setting, and the slanting rays made bands of sunlight and shadows, changing the colors of the flowers and meadows: bright where the light fell, and dull where the shadows were. The rays varied as the sun went down, and with it, the patterns in front of our eyes. It was like watching Monet or Van Gogh come to life. We stood in quiet awe, wrapped in each other's arms.

Ara always loved my recitation of Bengali and English poems. I had learned them on my own or in my school and college classes. Knowing that romantic and nature poems were her favorites, I was stirred to quote Wordsworth, one of my cherished English poets:

From: "Ode: Intimations of Immortality from Recollections of Early Childhood"

There was a time when meadow, grove, and stream,
The earth, and every common sight,
To me did seem
Apparelled in celestial light,
The glory and the freshness of a dream.
It is not now as it hath been of yore; —
Turn wheresoe'er I may,
By night or day.
The things which I have seen I now can see no more . . .

Though nothing can bring back the hour
Of splendour in the grass, of glory in the flower;
We will grieve not, rather find
Strength in what remains behind . . .

The scenes here took Ara and me back again to our early lives in our birthplace, the verdant tropical land—how much of nature's splendor we had witnessed. For the present, however, we couldn't disagree more with our revered poet. We still saw the freshness of the meadow, grove, and stream, and the celestial light. True, we couldn't bring back the hour, but the splendor in the grass and the glory in the flower were still intensely real to us. In that moment, we had no reason to grieve for whatever we had lost.

I was so absorbed in all this that I lost track of time. "Let's go, it's going to get dark," Ara said.

As much as I wanted to linger in this blissful landscape, I had to leave. She was more cautious than I. It's easy to take wrong turns in the dark on unmarked trails in the far country. This had happened to us once during another wildflower escapade. As we were going round and round in the dark trying to find a paved road, we saw a car coming toward us. We were frightened. If we got robbed, or worse, shot—almost everyone has guns in Texas and they are dead serious about protecting private property—no one would know. Fortunately, it was a game warden. He had seen our headlights from a distance and took us to be poachers of deer and other wildlife. After a stern warning, he showed us the way.

167

More than three years had gone by since Mrs. Cooper's disaster from her last chemo, and she was still in remission. She managed herself at her own home with the help of her daughter and granddaughter. She was ninety-one, but the sharpness of her mind had changed little.

One day, what we all dreaded happened. She fell in her bathtub and broke her bones—not an uncommon occurrence among the elderly. An ambulance brought her to the hospital.

The orthopedist who examined her didn't give us much hope. "Too many fractures in the hip, ribs, and arms," he said. "It's impractical to fix them all. And she won't survive long anesthesia and surgery."

She was placed in a nursing home, the very last place she wanted to be. When her husband had suffered from heart problems, his doctors suggested a nursing home for him, thinking that his old wife couldn't cope with the burden. But she kept him at their farmhouse until he died. Now she knew well that the days of her independence were gone forever. She had fought her cancer bravely and had lived on her own terms. But fate rules even the strongest of us.

Her pain was kept under control. When she was lucid, she was philosophical. "I've done what I could," she said once. "I've had a long life. I have to go sometime." Seeing my sadness, she said, "Is dying in the town any better than dying in the country?"

For the first time, Molly broke down. I consoled her as best I could. It was Susan who was stoic now. It seemed her grandmother's acute anguish during her last hospitalization was etched in her psyche.

Soon, Mrs. Cooper's pain became intractable. The nursing home was reluctant to dispense enough morphine. It was a dreaded drug for them, for morphine has the potential to cause respiratory arrest, especially in the elderly, and they worried about medical liability. But I insisted they give her as much as she needed. Still, she sometimes groaned in pain. In between, she hallucinated and said words that were demeaning to others and to herself. Though I should have known better, I was having difficulty seeing her reduced to this.

Susan took off from work to stay with her grandmother and care for her at the nursing home. One time she came to me, despondent. "Am I selfish, Dr. R?" she asked. "I want my grandmother to go. Is it because she's so difficult now?"

"You aren't selfish," I reassured her. "Because you love her, you don't want her to suffer."

One night, Mrs. Cooper was in particularly agonizing pain. She received the higher doses of morphine that I prescribed. Finally, she quieted down and went to sleep. She never woke up again.

I, like Molly and Susan, loved her dearly and, like them, I was grateful that she had left us.

Mrs. Cooper, like my grandmother, carved a lasting impression on me. My grandmother was an unlettered woman who lived in an isolated village her whole life. It was she who reproached me that collecting certificates alone wouldn't bring me wisdom. She had died a long time ago, and since then, I had indeed collected a lot of certificates in my career, but at times I wondered if I had met her expectations. In my earlier encounters with Mrs. Cooper, my ignorance made me blind to her intellect, because she lived outside my perception of culture and civilization.

Mrs. Cooper only had primary schooling; in her growing-up years, educating girls was thought to be a luxury. She spent her life from birth to death in farm country, away from cities. She and my grandmother came from entirely different continents and cultures, but they had something in common, something that gives meaning to life: wisdom. A new illumination from these two wise women sharpened my sight, and I now clearly saw what my grandmother meant: being schooled and gaining wisdom are not the same thing.

PART 5

JUAN: FOR TRUST AND DIGNITY

CHAPTER 19

He was a new referral to me. His doctor urged me to work him into my busy schedule, and I did so for the sake of a colleague. As I entered the exam room, he said in a testy tone, "Doctors have given me enough runaround. Looks like you're the same."

He was upset because I was late by about twenty minutes. I had been busy in the ICU trying to stabilize a chemo patient with sepsis.

"I'm sorry," I said, "I couldn't avoid the delay. The ICU took more time than I expected."

"I've seen quite a few doctors already. They always keep me waiting as if my time and me don't matter. But you're supposed to be different—that's what Dr. Allende told me."

This wasn't a good beginning with a new referral. I couldn't help but doubt my judgment in accepting him in a hurry for the sake of a friend. It wasn't that I had no idea about his temperament. Dr. Gabriela Allende, the young VA physician who had referred him, had cautioned me beforehand.

"He can be quite contrary," she said, sounding apologetic, "but his problem is beyond my expertise. That's why I need your help." She was a newcomer to a VA clinic that had opened recently.

I had been practicing for twenty years, and I had tried to be helpful to the new physicians. I hadn't forgotten how a few of the older doctors treated me when I began my practice—they were dismissive of me because of my background and my lack of experience. And generally, they disdained women and minority doctors, American-born or not.

"I've seen my share of contrary people," I laughed. This seemed to reassure her.

"Thank you for helping me out," she said in a more relaxed voice.

As I stood in the room, I sensed that the patient was more than contrary—he was trying to suppress his hostility toward me.

Juan Garcia was fifty-six years old. He had been treated at his regional VA hospital for cirrhosis of the liver. When he started to have new symptoms—discomfort in the right upper abdomen and right shoulder—he returned to his VA doctor. The doctor found that his liver was larger than before. An abdominal CT scan showed hepatic nodules. Since hepatic nodules are common in cirrhosis, the doctor decided to see him back for a follow-up before ordering further tests. (Hepatic comes from the Greek *hepar*, the liver.)

Juan's appetite became poorer as the days went by, and he was losing weight. When he went back to his VA hospital again, his doctor suspected something more serious than cirrhosis. Therefore, he sent him to a bigger VA hospital in Albuquerque, New Mexico, five hundred miles from his home in San Angelo, rather than to the VA hospital in San Antonio, only two hundred miles away. That's how the VA system operated then. Patients had to go to the designated referral centers, no matter how far, even when there was an equally good VA hospital closer to home.

A repeat abdominal CT scan in Albuquerque revealed the same liver changes as before.

"The doctors told me they couldn't do anything for cirrhosis," Juan said. "They thought I was still drinking, though I'd stopped drinking years ago."

After about three months, his abdominal discomfort and right shoulder pain got worse. This time, rather than returning to his VA hospital so far away, he went to the new VA clinic in San Angelo and saw Dr. Allende.

As I dug deeper, I realized his symptoms weren't from the cirrhosis alone. He didn't bring his medical records except the referral note. Dr. Allende had already told me that his records were scattered here and there, and it wouldn't be easy to pull them all together. But she gave me the information she had.

I asked Juan some questions to get a sense of his medical background.

"If I tell you the truth," he said, "you aren't going to like me. I know how doctors feel about drug addicts. Once you tell them about it, they don't trust and respect you anymore, even if you've been clean for a long time. But then they expect you to believe and follow whatever they say."

"I'll help you if I can."

My promise calmed him, and he became more forthcoming.

"I was drafted by the Army right after high school. They sent me to Vietnam.

I didn't fit in with any group until I finally found one that accepted me. I got into alcohol and drugs with them. I got hepatitis B in Vietnam. Later I came to my senses. I quit both alcohol and drugs after I was married at twenty-four."

His hepatitis B was most likely of the acute variety, not the chronic type, since it had resolved. He also admitted that he had missed two or three recent VA appointments. When I asked him why, he said, "Some of the doctors and nurses turned me off. Besides, I couldn't afford to go that far—gas costs money."

Despite his complaints, he wasn't against all VA hospitals. "I liked the Houston VA very much," he said. "I always kept my appointments there. They were good to me. I was working in an oil refinery in Port Arthur back then. It was just a ninety-minute drive from there."

Looking slightly withered, he had a shrunken face with stubble, but his hair was combed. He wore a clean brown shirt and blue jeans, and his shoes were weathered. It seemed he was trying to stay groomed but couldn't keep up because of his illness. I detected mild jaundice and an enlarged liver. He experienced pain in the right shoulder when he took a deep breath, but no symptoms whatsoever in his left shoulder.

I ordered labs and a CT of the abdomen and asked him to come back in a few days.

After Juan left, I was alone in my office that evening. Some patients reminded me of my past, and once in a while, I had a habit of ruminating about it. Juan brought back my memories of the Houston VA and my training at Baylor College of Medicine in the 1970s. Besides the VA, I rotated at BCM's other two main teaching hospitals, Methodist and Ben Taub General. At the time, it took me a while to get used to the wide disparities among these hospitals.

Methodist was one of the top hospitals in the country, a mecca of medicine, made famous by the giant Dr. Michael E. DeBakey. There, VIPs and royalty from around the world were regular patients. One of the most famous was Edward VIII, the ex-king of Britain and its empire, who, in 1936, abdicated the throne to marry an American divorcée, Wallis Simpson.

Ben Taub was the charity hospital of Harris County in Houston, the fourth-largest city in the US. It had the woes of a big-city charity hospital and housed the sick and the dying whom no other place wanted—poor minorities and destitute Whites. It wasn't easy to deal with Ben Taub's cancer patients amid its constant dire medical emergencies and its shortage of resources, resources that were taken for granted at Methodist. The distance between these two hospitals was less than a mile, but in reality, they were located on two different planets.[4]

The Houston VA hospital fell in between Methodist and Ben Taub when it came to patients. It was a big hospital and relatively calm. It wasn't without its problems, though. One of my greatest distresses came from its alcoholic patients. I had never witnessed such ravages of chronic alcoholism in one place. Many veterans said they had never recovered from the mental trauma of the battlefields. At the time, PTSD from war trauma was still more of a concept than a reality and wasn't taken seriously either by the medical profession or by the public. And right or wrong, some veterans who suffered from it found solace in alcohol.

The hospital was full of patients with cirrhosis of the liver, peripheral neuropathy, and alcoholic dementia. But more surprising for me was seeing the "third world" diseases, such as pellagra, caused by nicotinic acid deficiency, with its dermatitis, diarrhea, and mental disturbances; and scurvy from vitamin C deficiency, leading to bleeding gums, slow wound healing, anemia, and infection. The alcoholics' poor dietary habits and malnutrition were the reasons for the paucity of these vitamins. I had seen pellagra and scurvy among the destitute at Dhaka Medical College Hospital; those sufferers hadn't acquired their maladies from alcohol but rather from starvation as a result of being impoverished.

A large number of alcoholics at the VA hospital were also chronic smokers, and many presented with lung and head-neck cancers. Emphysema, diabetes, coronary disease, and stroke were common as well, as were peripheral circulatory problems. Some patients had gangrenous legs that required amputation. Those who had cancer on top of all this had a wretched existence.

Another painful experience came from the VA's urology ward. Dozens

---

4 Since my BCM training about fifty years ago, Ben Taub has transformed a great deal. Ricardo Nuila, a current Ben Taub doctor and a BCM professor, in his eloquent book, *The People's Hospital: Hope and Peril in American Medicine,* describes how Ben Taub is pioneering compassionate and yet less costly care compared to its rich neighboring nonprofit hospitals at the Texas Medical Center, the largest medical complex in the world for teaching and research. The Texas Medical Center includes, among more than sixty medical institutions, Ben Taub, Methodist, MD Anderson Cancer Center, Texas Children's Hospital, BCM, and the University of Texas Health Science Center.

of young men lay in their beds helplessly. They had paraplegia from spinal cord injury and had lost control of their bladders, so they required urinary catheters. They often had to battle catheter-related infections. After undergoing repeated antibiotic treatments, some of them had become resistant to common antibiotics. The most unfortunate ones also suffered from fecal incontinence, and despite the best efforts of the nurses, it wasn't easy to get rid of the foul smell.

Dejection and despair were written on the faces of these desperate men. I would have liked to know about their inner lives, but they were reticent to recount their nightmares. It seemed they were rationing whatever little strength they had been left with to cope with the present. What was the use of frittering it away on a past horror over which they had no control, then or now? They were the victims of the capricious whims of our political leaders, who instigated and supported a needless tragedy, the Vietnam War.

At times I got discouraged by my limitations, as I had at Dhaka Medical College Hospital. My efforts were scarcely making a difference in their daily lives. They would never get their legs back, nor would they void normally. They had no hope and no future, and I had no power to offer them either. After a while, whenever I got a consult from this ward, I felt an aversion to going there. Once, I used to be a big fan of war movies. They glorified heroic feats and sacrifices and romanticized daring actions happening in exotic, faraway lands. After my experience at the VA's urology ward, I lost my appetite for these films.

At first, I thought whatever ills had befallen Juan Garcia, at least he had managed to avoid the fate of those unfortunates. Once I reviewed his new abdominal CT, however, I realized the ill fate had followed him: he had masses in his liver that looked menacing. They were consistent with hepatocellular carcinoma (HCC) or hepatoma, one of the most lethal malignancies, killing 80 percent of patients within three years. But in reality, many of them lived barely eight months from the time of diagnosis. And the diagnosis itself had limitations like a few other malignancies, such as ovarian cancer, for the patients commonly remained asymptomatic until the disease had progressed quite far. (Note: The diagnosis and prognosis have been slowly improving in recent years.)

Hepatoma is a primary cancer of the liver, originating from the liver itself, and not a metastatic malignancy from another organ like the colon or breast.

Chronic hepatitis B and C and cirrhosis of the liver are the main causative factors. Juan had long-standing cirrhosis, but his hepatitis was apparently of the acute variety, though it was difficult to know for sure.

In the US, at present, the incidence of hepatoma is relatively low compared to cancers of the colon, breast, or lung. About 35,000 new hepatoma cases occur annually, and about 28,000 patients die from it. However, its incidence has been increasing over the last several decades. Since hepatitis C and chronic hepatitis B are its prime causes, the sheer number of these infections is frightening: about three to five million in the US. Another worrisome fact is that most of the infected persons are unaware of their infections. On top of this, the opioid crisis has been fueling the rise of hepatitis B.

These numbers have important public health significance. Since the incubation period between the hepatitis virus infections and hepatoma is between two and three decades, the tumor's prevalence and the resulting deaths will keep rising. The hope is that with the current effective hepatitis vaccines and better control of the opioid crisis, a potential epidemic could be averted.[5]

Because of Juan's abnormal CT, I tested for a hepatoma marker called alpha feto-protein (AFP). Normally, it's produced by the liver of a developing fetus. But due to the cancer's biological quirks, it's also made by hepatoma. Juan's AFP was high, supporting the CT finding.

Would I be justified giving him the fatal news without a biopsy confirmation, no matter how strongly my conclusion fit his case? I didn't think so, for he was only fifty-six, and a biopsy is the cardinal test for proving any malignancy. One way to do the biopsy was to insert a hollow needle through the skin into the liver mass, guided by CT, and taking a small sample of a lesion for pathologic examination.

My own decision would be useless without his consent, and to get it, I would have to tell him the unpleasant facts. Patients want truth, and it's truth that builds trust between doctors and patients. But conveying to him the reason for the biopsy wouldn't be easy. He felt alienated by doctors and distrusted them, and I was still trying to earn his trust. But what had to be done, had to be done.

---

5 The issue also has global importance. On the continents with the fastest growing populations—Africa and Asia—hepatitis of various forms is endemic. Hence, hepatoma is among the commonest malignancies, and worldwide, annually, more than a million patients die of it, with the attendant medical and social costs. So making progress on hepatitis and its consequences will benefit all humanity.

CHAPTER 20

I planned to introduce the biopsy to Juan slowly to weigh his reaction, then go from there. But as soon as he saw me, he asked bluntly, "What's the matter with me that so many doctors can't figure it out?"

"I may have the answer for you."

"Are you sure?"

"Not completely, but if you give me a chance I can be sure."

I told him about the CT and the need for the liver biopsy, and why Albuquerque wanted him for a follow-up that he missed. He may have had some inkling about possible cancer from Dr. Allende since she had referred him to me, an oncologist, rather than to a liver specialist. He didn't raise any arguments about my points.

He looked at me intently and asked, "If you find cancer, can you take care of it?"

I hesitated, but I had to let him know.

"Surgery is the best treatment, but your liver tumors are too numerous for that. A new medicine has come out, though. I don't know how well it'll work."

"What's the use of the biopsy then?"

"To confirm the diagnosis and give the medicine a try. It's up to you."

"I need to find out. I'm tired of sickness."

I preferred to get his family involved before the biopsy. He had told me before that his wife had died and he lived alone. She'd been on dialysis for four years due to kidney failure from diabetes and hypertension. "I did all I could for her. We were married for thirty-two years. I wish she were with me."

He then said more about his family. "I have a daughter and a son. She lives near Houston. I can't bother her; she has a hard enough life. She's divorced

179

with three small children and works as a nurse's aide. My son lives in Big Spring. He's on his own, works for an oil company."

"Would you bring him to talk about things together?"

"We don't agree on things, but I'll try."

A few days later, Juan came in with his son, Alberto, a handsome man in his mid-twenties. Unlike his father, he was polished. I was so anxious to establish a connection with Juan that I had waited to ask him two very personal questions, because they were related to his drug abuse. I couldn't wait any longer if I was going to schedule him for the biopsy. His answers would dictate whether any special precautions would be necessary for an invasive procedure. But how could I bring up these questions in front of Alberto?

"I need to talk to your dad in private for a minute," I said to Alberto. "Would you mind sitting in my office? I'll call you back soon."

Juan interrupted. "Let him stay, you can ask me whatever you want."

"It may embarrass you both."

"I have an idea what you'll ask. It's about time we bring it out."

"Have you had an HIV test?"

Alberto's eyes went wide as he looked at his father.

"Yes," Juan said without hesitation. "The VA hospital did it, and they didn't find anything."

"The next question is more personal, Juan. It's better if Alberto goes out."

"No, he's an adult now," Juan said emphatically. "He needs to know what his father has done. It's easier for me if it comes out here."

"Have you had multiple sexual partners since the HIV test?"

His son reacted sharply. "What does his sex life have to do with his liver trouble? Are you insulting my father because he comes from the VA?"

"No, HIV information is essential, VA or not," I said.

Juan glanced at his son and then looked at me and said, "The other day, Dr. Allende at the VA clinic checked it again. She said it's all right."

"Why would you have an HIV test now, Dad?" Alberto asked him. "You've been off the drugs for so long."

"Well, you know, I've been lonely since your mother died."

Then he turned his head towards the wall and said, "I took precautions."

I sensed that tension had developed between the father and son after the death of the young man's mother. With Juan's future at stake, perhaps for the sake of reconciliation, he wanted his son to know all about his past.

Finally, we came to the main topic: the biopsy. Alberto inquired if his father had other options.

The patient answered for himself, aiming at me. "I'll get the biopsy and settle the matter. At least you've taken me seriously like Dr. Allende. This is one of the few times I've gotten straight answers."

Alberto rolled his eyes and burst out, "He's always done things his own way. I don't matter to him." Then, as he stood up to leave, he added, "He's a hard man to know, and I'm his son."

The radiologists did all the needle biopsies in the x-ray department since they were guided by CT. I asked the radiologist who routinely performed liver biopsies to do Juan's procedure.

"I didn't read his CT," he said. He brought the films from the x-ray files and put them on the view box. He scanned it for a few minutes, then pointed his finger at the liver and said, "Look how much cirrhosis he's got—he's a poor risk for biopsy."

"His liver function tests are within the satisfactory range," I said, and gave him the results. "You can see, clinically he's really an average risk."

He waved his hands. "I'd rather not take a chance."

He had denied a few of my other patients before because they were "poor risks." I had noticed that my patients he determined were "poor risks" were either Blacks or Hispanics. Whether his refusals were chance happenings or something else, I didn't know.

I then went to another radiologist, a friend I'll call Dr. S. He was also accomplished in needle biopsies, but he had more experience with kidneys and lungs.

"I'll help you out," he said, and he did help.

Dr. S finished the biopsy, with no complications. Pathology confirmed HCC—that is, hepatoma.

I called Dr. Allende at the VA clinic. "Gabriela, I have unfortunate news for Juan Garcia."

She heard me out and said, "I was afraid of that. This could've been diagnosed earlier. I've gotten some of his old records now. They mentioned his being a noncompliant, unreliable patient, and speculated he was still drinking."

She then gave me her own observations. "He isn't the easiest patient, I know. But the doctors and nurses became unfairly fixated on his drug and alcohol abuse, so it was easy to label him as unreliable and noncompliant."

Juan himself had mentioned to me the words "trust" and "dignity." Patients or not, we all yearn for trust and dignity.

Gabriela raised a pertinent issue: patients' compliance and the labels we use, fairly or unfairly. From my own experience, I have understood the factors for noncompliance. A few patients indeed are irresponsible and don't take part in their own care; they go to doctors only when they have no other recourse. Other patients, however, are disenchanted with the system, and this starts with the doctors and nurses, some of whom disdain addicts and alcoholics and look at them with suspicion, especially if they are illiterate and poor. In turn, these patients come to distrust doctors and hospitals. At Methodist, the medical mecca, we treated with courtesy any drunken executive brought to the ER. But the once-drinking patients at Ben Taub, the charity hospital, received quite the opposite reception, and it followed them even after they had quit alcohol years before. A few other groups are noncompliant due to handicaps. They have unresolved psychiatric problems, or are trapped by their practical difficulties, like traveling long distances or having no social support.

I discussed with Gabriela how to manage hepatocellular carcinoma and its constraints.

"I'll leave it to your judgment," she said. "But if Juan needs chemotherapy, I'd have to clear it through the VA system first."

I explained that doxorubicin had been used with marginal results. In any case, with Juan, its benefit would not outweigh its toxicity. But there was a new drug for HCC called Nexavar that I wanted Juan to try. It belonged to the new class of drugs called TKIs. (TKIs have been elaborated on in part 3 with J. D. and his CML.)

"Nexavar is a tablet," I added, "and though it has its own side effects, it's still more tolerable than doxorubicin."

"Any idea about its cost?" she asked.

Her concern was valid—prior approval wasn't easy for any expensive drug, and a new one at that.

"I'll check and let you know."

I found out Nexavar's cost. Oncologists are used to high-priced medicines—how could I forget the price of Gleevec? Still, I was again shocked to learn that a month's supply of Nexavar was a whopping $21,000. Its dose was four tablets daily, so each tablet cost $174, giving a daily total of $696. On top of that was the added cost of the antinausea medications.

This was the Nexavar price in the United States, so I got curious to know what it was in Canada, their medical care being equivalent to ours. What a surprise! Nexavar was selling at only a quarter of the US price: $44 a tablet, for a monthly total of $5,280. This was one more example of how US patients were gouged to the hilt, with no reprieve in sight. Moreover, the out-of-pocket costs are increasing year by year. Again, to quote Hagop Kantarjian of MD Anderson: "Traditional free-market forces are not working well in healthcare."

I informed Dr. Allende what I had discovered about the cost of Nexavar.

"We're just a new clinic," she said. "It's going to be difficult to do much from here. Let me refer him to one of the big city VA hospitals."

Juan was aghast at the expense, as I was. Moreover, he wasn't ready to go to another VA location. He realized, however, that Gabriela and I were trying to help him out, and we didn't have endless time to argue. He relented and took Gabriela's advice.

Juan returned to me two weeks later, angry, and feeling worse than before. His abdominal pain had increased, and he was eating less and losing more weight. Also worrisome, despite taking analgesics, he was having trouble sleeping at night because of the worsening shoulder pain with breathing.

Why was his pain worrisome even though he had no metastasis there? It was because of its peculiar nature, known as "referred pain," a common symptom in hepatoma caused by the involvement of the phrenic nerve. This nerve begins in the neck and then passes down the shoulder to each side of the diaphragm to control its breathing movements (*phrenic* means related to the diaphragm). Since the liver is located under the right dome of the diaphragm, as the hepatoma grows, it irritates the dome and its phrenic nerve, which, in turn, sends the pain signal to the right shoulder, resulting in the shoulder pain with breathing.

To persuade Juan to go to the VA for his medicine, I had told him that once the tumor shrank with Nexavar, both his abdominal and shoulder pain would improve. I thought he had already begun the treatment, and it was too early to expect a response.

"They didn't give me the medicine," he said. "They want *you* to write the prescription. One of the nurses told me that if they wrote the prescription, they'd have to give me the Nexavar and it would come out of their own budget."

It was understandable that a VA hospital, like any other organization, operated within a defined budget, but this flagrant rationing was new to me. There must be a way to make exceptions for a veteran like Juan with a life-and-death matter.

Juan added, "Talking to them, I felt like they saw no chance for me, so why waste money? They asked me to come home and ask our VA clinic to find a hospice. I know my cancer is bad, but I'm not about to die. Why should I go to a hospice? Don't I deserve treatment first?"

I tried to tell him that he still needed the VA's help and I wasn't a VA doctor. But he was impatient with me. "I've heard enough excuses. Are you giving me the prescription, or are you going to do like them?"

I called Dr. Allende again and told her what had transpired.

"Please write him the prescription," she urged. "I'll do my best to get it approved quickly. He can't afford to buy it himself."

He took my prescription to Gabriela. I was relieved that this time he would get Nexavar started.

Four days later, I got a call from a VA pharmacist. "We can't fill this prescription," he said. "You've written the wrong dose."

"It's not the wrong dose," I clarified. "The patient's liver is abnormal, and since Nexavar is metabolized by the liver, he may not be able to handle the full dose at first. So, I want him to start with 50 percent of the dose. If he can tolerate it, we'll raise it to the standard amount."

The pharmacist wasn't satisfied. "We need a letter certifying that. Otherwise, we can't honor the prescription."

Juan's son telephoned me not long after my conversation with the VA pharmacist. He, too, was upset. "The least you could do was to give my father the right dose. Are you trying to save money for the VA because he's a Mexican American?"

"No, it's not that at all, Alberto. I told the reason for the lower dose to your dad when I gave him the prescription."

"He didn't say anything to me about this."

"You know, he's sick and under a lot of stress. He probably forgot to mention it to you at the time."

"I still don't understand him. I'm sorry I've bothered you."

I may also have told Juan too much about Nexavar's metabolism to justify my dosing. By now, I should have mastered what was too much or too little when it came to informing patients. My shortfall hit me in the face when I read what Jeri Dyson, a doctor and cancer survivor, had to say about her own experience: "I'm a physician, and I was having difficulty processing the seemingly endless amount of information my oncologist was hurtling at me. I wondered how patients without a medical degree handled all the information presented to them at diagnosis."

To simplify things for Juan, I should have written the standard dose and then asked him to start with half the amount. But I didn't want to take any chances in case he followed the written instructions on the medicine bottle. Whatever good intentions I had seemed to matter little.

A senior colleague once gave me advice on how to handle rules and regulations: "Don't try to fight them too much if you want to avoid burnout. It's easier if you learn how to play the game." I thought then that it was a cop-out not to resist the mindless policies. But after encountering roadblocks again and again, I realized how right he was. The unpredictable regulations were hard to keep up with, and they came from all directions: hospitals, insurance companies, Medicare and Medicaid, Tricare, with the VA thrown into the mix.

To further complicate things, the cancer field was changing fast—new diagnoses and treatments and new equipment were coming at us full speed. The computerization of medicine to make it more efficient was on the rise and proved to be not as useful as touted. Novel computer programs were constantly being introduced. No sooner had you finished spending hours learning one program than another was promoted in the name of—you guessed it—improvement, and you had to go through a whole new round of training again. It felt like a never-ending cycle.

To add to the difficulty, when doctors followed hospitalized patients, often they didn't talk to the patients' nurses directly, as done previously; instead, doctors went to the computer and read their entries. In the process, patient care became more and more impersonal. All this, not just witnessing suffering and death and dying, led to physician burnout.

I, like many, believe that practicing medicine is more of an art than a science. Computer screens give you tons of scientific data and facts, but not the judgment needed to sift through the data to meet the needs of an individual patient—that's the art of medicine. Moreover, in the clutter, what's essential can get lost.

I decided to take the easy way out with Juan. I wasn't going to justify my dosing by writing a clarifying letter. That would generate more correspondence, which would delay his treatment. I simply gave him a new prescription with the regular dosage and firmly asked him to take half of the daily dose until he saw me in two weeks.

I wished the VA wasn't this tangled. I waited with anxiety and hoped for the best for Juan.

CHAPTER 21

D r. Allende's persistence paid off and Juan got his medicine. He tolerated the first round of the low-dose Nexavar with no significant discomfort. As his abdominal and shoulder pain lessened, he began to feel better. With time, little by little, the progress was additive. He could eat more, and his weight loss stopped. Also important, his alpha feto-protein marker was lower than before. Everything taken together, the medicine was reducing his tumor. Another good thing was that myelosuppression wasn't an issue with Nexavar.

Alberto, Juan's son, was concerned that his father wasn't eating a balanced diet and that he was consuming too much junk food like French fries.

"Any eating is better than no eating all," I told him. "He needs calories first. We can think about the balance later." Pushing for "good food" when patients are anorectic and averse to meals is a fruitless exercise; this also aggravates them when their lives are already full of frustration.

My experience with diet during my bout with kala-azar, which almost extinguished my life, had been imprinted on me; this was after my mother's death when I was only seven. I became shrunken and pot-bellied from my huge liver and spleen caused by the parasitic illness. I was nauseated and ano-rectic from the intensely bitter medicine mixtures, and I resisted food. My doctor's insistence on a proper diet did me no good. Seeing my sorry state, my older brother, Bazlur, ignored the rules and saved me with what little food I accepted, good or bad. With this, I was able to handle the medicine and slowly improved and was able to eat more. My despair dissolved and I graduated to a balanced diet that helped me to overcome the illness. That's why I followed my brother's dietary philosophy for some of my chemotherapy patients.

After some time, I raised Juan's dose to three tablets daily. His symptoms ameliorated further, and he gained weight. After three months, I got VA permission for a follow-up CT. A great relief—Juan had achieved partial remission (PR), which is regression of a tumor by 50 percent or more. (A complete remission, or CR, is the disappearance of all tumors, primary or metastatic.)

Some cancers can have long partial remission with treatment, with a good quality of life, while others develop resistance and spread with a vengeance. I was afraid of taking a risk with hepatoma, and I hoped that with the standard dose, Juan would have less chance of failure and more chance of CR or at least a durable PR.

So I raised the dose to 4 tablets (800 mg) daily. In about a week, he developed diarrhea and fatigue. As if these weren't bad enough, he became the casualty of a toxicity called Hand-Foot Syndrome, which causes pain and swelling of the palms and soles of the feet.

His functioning that had been improving so far decreased sharply, and his spirits sank. The standard dose was too much for him; his threshold was 600 mg, since he had tolerated that amount fairly well. Therefore, we returned to 600 mg. His diarrhea and fatigue receded, as did the pain and swelling of his extremities. So much for the "standard" dose—what's standard for one is toxic for another. After all, chemo and Nexavar and the like are still imprecise forms of remedy.

While we maintained the daily dose of 600 mg, Dr. Allende patiently smoothed our way through the VA labyrinth. We did Juan's third CT in six months. His tumor had shrunk further, though not as much as before. This kind of response is a common theme. Not all the cells in a cancer are the same, for they have their life cycles and are in all stages of development and maturation. Some cells respond to therapy better than others. The cells that are most sensitive to chemo are killed first, so the tumor shrinks faster in the beginning. More recalcitrant cells die slowly and delay the tumor regression. Juan's alpha feto-protein, the hepatoma marker, however, was much lower.

The radiologist who had refused to do Juan's liver biopsy reviewed his CT this time. His kind of reasoning was familiar to me.

"I went by hepatoma's overall survival rate," he said. "I didn't think he was going to make its median eight months and would be lucky to last around three months. But the last two CTs indicate he may go longer than that. Sorry, Fazlur, I wasn't helpful."

While we were discussing Juan, an internist colleague happened by. He overheard what we were talking about. "Those VA headaches," he remarked, "with all their diabetes, hypertension, cirrhosis, and bad heart and lungs? I try to stay away from them."

He boasted that he didn't accept VA patients because, in his opinion, they were looking for free medicine, and they took too much time with their multisystem diseases. He was saying something openly that quite a few other doctors felt and practiced.

This being West Texas, most of these physicians were strongly conservative politically and supported the wars in Iraq and Afghanistan. Our private doctors' dining room was an illuminating place for exposing all sorts of ideas. National and world affairs were often a part of our debates. Ironically, there was a clear dichotomy in what some of these doctors championed and what they did for veterans.

"What's your obligation to these patients if you like war so much?" I had asked these colleagues.

"We live in a free country, we have a right to refuse anyone," was a common reply. "We don't believe in socialized medicine."

"What about the emergency room patients?"

"We see them because we're required by law."

But those vocal war proponents didn't limit their policy to VA patients only; they also applied it to the men and women on active duty. We have a military base in our city, and over the years, some of my colleagues and I had taken care of many soldiers and officers. The active-duty service members and their families were covered by a health insurance plan called Tricare. The vocal doctors refused to honor Tricare as well, since it reimbursed less than private insurances did. In fact, one overtly patriotic medical group ironically didn't accept Tricare patients at all.

Cancer treatment is a multidisciplinary endeavor. Patient management depends on doctors of many specialties, including primary care physicians, surgeons, medical and radiation oncologists, radiologists, and pathologists. But the physicians are only one part of the team; there are others who are also essential: nurses, pharmacists, technicians, social workers, and mental health professionals. There are still others who are not formal professionals, such as the nurse's aides and the manual workers who clean the hospital rooms to keep them hygienic and infection free.

Hospitals have a tumor board, which meets weekly to monthly to discuss the management of selected cancer cases, especially the complex ones. At our hospital, the professional team on the tumor board consisted of doctors, nurses, pharmacists, and social workers. At one of our tumor board meetings, we presented two entirely different patients: Juan Garcia and a twenty-six-year-old man named Buddy.

Buddy was a married father of two young children. He was a roustabout for a small oil company. He did what roustabouts do in the oil fields, hard physical labor amid the elements of nature—heat, freezing cold, rain, and dust storms. He worked where one couldn't avoid inhaling polluted air. Buddy was a conscientious employee and was willing to learn, and he worked a lot of overtime to better his family's means, for these jobs had low pay. His supervisor was pleased with his performance and had marked him for a promotion with higher wages.

After some time, however, Buddy's performance flagged. He felt weak and drained, and he blamed this on his long work hours. He cut down on his overtime, but it made no difference. His company, like some small outfits then, provided no health insurance and offered only what was mandated by law: workers' compensation coverage for job-related injuries. Being without health insurance, he couldn't afford to see a doctor. Soon, he began to lose weight and had a fever and a cough. At the insistence of his wife, he finally went to a walk-in clinic and paid in cash. The doctor diagnosed bronchitis and gave him an antibiotic.

But he got weaker, and drenching night sweats soaked his shirts. He missed work several times. These manual workers were easily disposable, and regardless of his stellar past, Buddy was fired.

His cough worsened and his breathing became labored, so his wife took him to the ER. A chest x-ray suggested a mass in the mediastinum, a space between the two lungs. A CT scan confirmed the mass. Its biopsy revealed Hodgkin's disease (HD), a cancer of the lymphocytes, a type of white cells. The cause of his symptoms—fever, night sweats, and weight loss—became clear. They were characteristic of Hodgkin's disease. (The disease is named after a British pathologist, Thomas Hodgkin, who first described it in 1832. It's now called Hodgkin's lymphoma.)

The merits and demerits of treatments were regularly argued at the tumor board, but this time, a heated debate ensued about the management of Buddy and Juan. A few members beat around the bush on the subject, rather than saying outright what they meant. Eventually, a surgeon, Dr. W, cut through the fog.

"Here you have a fifty-six-year-old unemployed man from the VA. His hepatoma is incurable, yet you're spending more than $20,000 a month on him. Then you have a young man in the prime of his life, whose Hodgkin's disease is curable. How do you justify this kind of misapplication of funds?"

To fortify his point, Dr. W reminded me about J. D., my patient with chronic myeloid leukemia, whom I had presented to this board in the past. At the time, I had bemoaned that though Gleevec had put J. D. into remission, he'd been compelled to stop it because of its high cost. He had lost his job and his health insurance along with it, and he couldn't afford to buy Gleevec on his own. As a result, his CML relapsed and transformed into acute leukemia, which required expensive, protracted treatment.

Dr. W was succinct in his conclusion: "The hepatoma money could have been used productively for patients like J. D. and Buddy."

His opinion seemed heartless, but it wasn't without merit. This sort of triage dilemma is brought up often, especially when it comes to pricey treatments for those with alcoholism and addiction, and who are considered callous about their own health.

I was, of course, fully cognizant of the costs and circumstances. As we had discussed before, a proven chemotherapy that cured advanced HD like Buddy's was MOPP. To reiterate, MOPP consists of nitrogen mustard, Oncovin, procarbazine, and prednisone; the first two are given IV and the second two are taken orally. MOPP costs less than Nexavar. In other words, Buddy's cancer could be cured at a lower cost, giving him a chance for a productive life, while Juan had no hope of a cure even with the higher cost.

Economic and ethical pronouncements, however, are easier to make when you are not at the patient's bedside. I was expected to answer the surgeon. Besides being an oncologist, I was the chair of the tumor board, so I had an additional responsibility to address the cancer issues.

But before I had a chance to speak, Dr. F, a family physician, raised his hand. I had worked with both Dr. F and the surgeon closely, and both were successful in their own fields. However, Dr. F, like most family physicians, earned only half of what the surgeon did. The latter, like many high earners, had a tendency to look down on the lower earners and saw them only as referral sources. (Higher income and prestige are the main reasons medical students aspire to become specialists and avoid family practice.)

"Sure, the cost-benefit calculation is important," the family physician said. "But if someone comes to me for help, I take care of her or him the best way I know how, regardless of the background. I choose an optimum treatment, and if it has a cheaper equivalent, I use that. I understand that in Juan Garcia's case, Nexavar happens to be the right drug, with no equivalent cheaper alternative."

He then turned to Buddy's case. "The young man raises fundamental questions in medicine for which we all are accountable. The cost of care is only one. Had he been covered by insurance, his diagnosis and treatment would've been completed earlier, and his suffering and work interruption would've been less. So how come we don't take a stand on access to care? Whatever faults Juan Garcia had, he had nothing to do with Buddy's access."

The family physician had hit a tender spot, for he was alluding to universal coverage, which some saw as socialized medicine, an idea they detested. They adhered to the obsolete notions of the past American Medical Association, which had adamantly opposed Medicare. (As a result, the once all-powerful AMA ultimately became a lesser force in medicine because of its refusal to change with the times.)

In our milieu, Dr. W, the conservative, had plenty of supporters. But several in the group came to Dr. F's defense. Then, an oncology nurse asked, "Is rationing for patients like Juan Garcia justified?"

This time, the family physician's partner spoke out. He looked at the surgeon, as if he, and not the nurse, had asked the question.

"Before we consider rationing, we must admit that we do too many tests, x-rays, and scans that don't benefit our patients." Then he raised his voice and added, "More important, we do too many costly, unnecessary surgeries. According to a 2010 CDC report, 51 million in-patient surgeries are done annually in the US, and close to that number of outpatient procedures. But the sad fact is that 10–20 percent of these procedures are unwarranted."

Having the chair's privilege, I let him go on, because it was clear that he and his partner were prepared to confront the topic while confronting the surgeon, and that they had studied the matter in depth.

"Let's take a specific example from a 2011 *JAMA* study. Out of 112,000 implantable cardioverter-defibrillators, 22.5 percent—that's more than 25,000—weren't indicated. Another study showed that out of 1.3 million cesarean sections per year, 130,000 were deemed unjustified. The same with spinal fusion and hysterectomy. Besides, these operations have their share of complications, which add to the enormous costs. They even cause disability and death."

Then, he was emphatic: "We must stop our own plague before we bring up the rationing question."

The surgeon stayed silent. But Ms. P, the head nurse of oncology, asked me, "Will you continue active treatment on Juan Garcia, no matter what?"

Ms. P was an experienced bedside nurse, and I had a great deal of respect for her. I felt that with her question, she was giving me an opening to explain myself.

"No, at a certain point I'll have to stop active intervention, as I would with any other patient. If his cancer becomes refractory to treatment, I'll ask for hospice."

We had gone overtime with all our arguments, and everyone needed to return to work. I decided to resume the discussion next time and adjourned the meeting.

Juan managed to have a fairly active life with Nexavar and volunteered at a hospital. He became good at dealing with cancer patients and spent time at their bedside. Pretty soon, he became known for his work, and that uplifted him.

This went on for fourteen more months, bringing his survival to two years. One morning, while he was driving to the hospital, his car was hit from the side by a driver who ignored a red light. Juan's abdominal pain recurred. He thought the pain was due to the accident, but rather than subsiding, it got worse. An abdominal CT revealed the most disconcerting news. The liver masses that had shrunk with treatment were bigger now. The inevitable had happened—Nexavar had stopped working. Pretty soon, the tumor ran wild, and pain confined Juan to bed.

Hospice was ideal to make his remaining days as easy as possible, but he had declined it when the VA first suggested it. What would I do if he refused it again?

CHAPTER 22

J uan knew he was at the end of the road. "I guess this is it, Dr. R," he said. "Now the VA can save their money."

"I realize you don't like hospice," I said, "but it's the best option we have now for keeping you comfortable."

"How do you know I don't like hospice?"

"Well, you were quite unhappy when the VA hospital recommended it."

"Just let me die without trying anything at all? I've had my chance—I don't mind hospice now."

Juan's home was in a barrio of the town. I went to see him a few times. He lived in a small two-bedroom house. His son and daughter-in-law came to help him whenever they could. A few of Juan's neighbors also extended their hands. An old grandmother in her seventies, who had her own family to look after, was particularly attentive to him and worked with the hospice nurses and aides. She was a devout woman from Juan's church. "Good or bad, I don't know," she told me, "but he's God's child like I am."

This was something that I had seen on quite a few occasions. Sometimes friends and neighbors and seeming strangers are more generous than family members. The former do things out of their good hearts, not for any self-interest or financial gain. Family members, on the other hand, are more apt to be alienated for one reason or another, often due to some form of discord about money and property. Besides, relatives or not, some humans are simply cold-hearted beings, and others' suffering means little to them.

One day I found Juan in a reflective mood. "My wife was the one who kept up with our family and neighbors. After she was gone, I kept to myself. I felt lost and aimless without her. I'm lucky my neighbors haven't forgotten me. I did what I could when I was healthy and I enjoyed my work. I regret my days with addiction and alcohol."

"We all make mistakes," I said. "We all have our strengths and weakness in one form or another."

In about two months, his eyes and skin became markedly yellow from the deepening jaundice, which meant his liver was failing badly. His hepatoma was growing fast and was devouring the whole liver. Soon, he became confused from hepatic encephalopathy, a disorder of the brain caused by buildup of toxins in the blood, toxins that are normally cleared by the liver. In a few days he went into what's called hepatic coma from complete liver failure—the level of toxins was too much for his brain. The coma ended in his everlasting sleep.

Juan's life and medical story, too, were instructive to me. Sometimes our past follows us and haunts us. Regardless, it was unfair for some doctors and nurses to get blinded by his past. He deserved dignity and trust, as the rest of us do. Whatever he was or was not, he was a patient after all and came to us for help.

Then, there's another side of VA medicine that we must look at: its image, as seen by the medical profession and the public, needs to change. Throughout my decades of training and practicing, most of my colleagues saw VA doctors and nurses as "second class." I had worked with VA doctors and their patients over the years, and I knew they wanted to do good for their patients, but often, tangled bureaucracy and a shortage of resources thwarted them. Sure, there were a few indifferent people at the VA, but indifferent people were outside the VA as well. The responsibility for improving VA medicine belongs to both the medical profession and society as a whole. We can't have one type of care for veterans and another for the rest of us.

Depending on the distance and scheduling of the funeral services of my patients, I was able to attend some of them. Like any medical oncologist, death was my frequent companion, so I had to be careful with my timetable. Irrespective of my deep feeling for the dead, I avoided doing things at the expense of the living under my care.

These funeral rites were enlightening to me as a doctor. I was, at times, wrong about the patients I thought I knew well. Of course, we always speak reverently of the departed in their final hours on the earth, regardless of their qualities, redeeming or not. Even then, you find out who they really were—and you may be surprised by the new revelations. Moreover, on occasion, you also learn something about the persons who eulogize them.

I had taken care of a surgical colleague in his early forties, Dr. D. So I got to know him both as a patient and as a doctor. He was a friendly, outgoing man, well liked by his patients, colleagues, and nurses. "He's easy to work with," the operating room nurses would tell me, "and his surgical complications are below the average." It says a lot about a surgeon when you hear this kind of compliment. The nurses who work with the doctors, day in and day out, under trying conditions, can judge them better than anyone else.

Dr. D was a busy surgeon with a large practice, and over the years, he had referred me many breast cancer patients for their chemotherapy. You can tell of the finesse of a surgeon's hands from observing ordinary findings, like post-op scars, and the scars on his mastectomy patients were far less disfiguring than those from other surgeons.

I admired his easygoing personality and his sense of humor to defuse tension. During our lunch hours at the doctors' dining room, we would often sit together at a corner table and talk about our families and patients, and about our common outside interests: arts and literature. We both loved Gabriel García Márquez and Pablo Neruda, except that he read them in their original Spanish, Spanish being his mother tongue, and I read them in their English translations. "There're some good translations all right," he would say, "but they can't fully grasp the nuances of the original."

Late one night, my home phone rang. I was groggy as I picked up the receiver. There was a sobbing sound on the other end, and I immediately became alert. It was my secretary, and she spoke haltingly in between her sobs. "Dr. D . . . Dr. D . . . shot himself. His nurse . . . his nurse just called me."

"Is he all right?" I was abrupt.

She hesitated and then said, "They brought him to the ER. The doctors couldn't revive him. I'm sorry, sir; you two were such good friends."

I was numb, trying to process the news and remembering Dr. D's final interaction with me. Just a few hours previously, I had asked him for a favor. I had a patient in the ICU who was deathly ill with bleeding and infection. I needed an intravenous catheter in a hurry to start antibiotics and blood transfusion. I called Dr. D: "You need to put in a Groshong line for me right now. I know you aren't on call, but I would rather have you do it."

He sensed the urgency in my voice. "Don't worry, I'm coming" he said. He did, and he finished the procedure without delay. Thanks to him, the patient pulled through.

His words, "Don't worry, I'm coming," kept buzzing in my ears. There must be a mistake; I was in a daze. A few minutes passed, and then the gravity of Dr. D's ending hit me. I jumped out of bed.

"What's the matter?" Ara asked as she switched on the bedside light. As a cancer doctor's wife, she was used to her husband's midnight calls. I didn't feel like talking. She had seen me somber whenever I had lost a patient with whom I had a close bond. "I have to go to the hospital," I said.

"Pay attention to your driving." Her usual admonition each time I left home at odd hours. It wasn't always easy for her, either.

After a while, the hospital CEO reached out to me. "I need your help, Dr. Rahman," he said. "I understand you're consulting on a few of Dr. D's patients in the hospital. Would you round on them until the other surgeons take over his cases? He was the current surgical chief, so we also need to appoint a temporary chief. Who do you think would be best?"

Hospital administrators don't ask for favors without reason. Losing Dr. D was upsetting for him on several counts. Dr. D was a star surgeon and a top revenue generator, and the hospital had enthusiastically promoted him to the public. Now, the hospital's star had become a public relations nightmare. The morning paper had a front-page headline on the suicide. I was amazed how quickly the newspaper had smelled the tragedy.

I wasn't the only one numbed by the sudden loss—the suicide had sent a shock wave all through the clinic and the hospital. Everyone was walking around downcast, and the atmosphere was hushed.

Dr. D's funeral service was held at his church in a poor part of the town; though he had moved to an affluent neighborhood, he never abandoned his old house of worship. The church was packed with mourners. Many had dripping eyes. A young underling of the priest conducted the service. I felt sorry for him—he tried hard not to use the word "suicide," but he was not yet good at concocting convoluted language. I heard that the old priest himself had refused to come. I wondered what happened to Dr. D's special status—in Dr. D's earthly life, the cleric considered him a valued member of the congregation. My friend was moral when he lived but apparently became immoral because of his manner of death. Would he have gotten even this little grace if he hadn't been a doctor?

There were only two eulogizers, and after they finished, Dr. D's wife, Alma, stood up. All eyes gazed at her. She walked to the podium, head held high. The people around me traded surprised looks. I, too, was puzzled. She wasn't on the list of speakers.

Turning to the audience, she said, "My husband was a good man, you all know." Her voice was clear. "He worked so hard to build a career. He was dedicated to his patients. I supported him all the way, but it seems I didn't do enough for him." She choked up.

After she composed herself, she pushed aside her prepared script. Her voice turned stern as she talked, and she used some Spanish words and sentences for emphasis. "Some are saying that God has taken him away for His own reasons. I don't believe that. *Dios no se lo llevó a él, el Diablo lo hizo.*" I understood some Spanish, and I knew *diablo* meant devil. But why would she bring up the devil now? And what did it have to do with Dr. D? While I was trying to comprehend the rest of the sentence, she translated it herself. "God didn't take him, the devil did." Then she added, "Don't forget that the devil can also possess any of you just as it possessed my husband." All this thoroughly astonished me.

Some in the congregation were my friends or had been my patients. I looked in all directions. I sensed that they weren't used to hearing this kind of bluntness from a layperson, especially from a woman, and in such a solemn circumstance. The men and women seemed embarrassed, and even afraid of what she might say next. She raised her voice further and said, "*Y ese diablo es la depresión descontrolada.* [And that devil is uncontrolled depression.]"

I had known Alma for almost as long as I had known her husband. She was a beautiful, graceful woman with a melodious voice. But this wasn't the same person.

She continued. "I ask you to be careful. The same *diablo* can easily destroy you." She took a deep breath as she surveyed the crowd and repeated, "*El diablo, la depresión.*"

Then she became more intimate and told us how Dr. D had tried hard to fight his depression by himself and had refused to seek professional help. He was worried that if the matter got out, it would hurt his practice. He had gone through many struggles and a great deal of personal sacrifice to become a surgeon. He came from a poor family. He had reached the crest of his career, and he didn't want to let his loved ones down or let his colleagues and patients lose faith in him.

Now that Alma had made her point, I thought she would stop there. But she didn't, and she tackled a subject that was anathema.

"Our *machismo* culture also played a part in his resistance," she said. "As if openly admitting depression is beneath one's own macho image. If I sound harsh, it's because I want to. We struggled so hard to get to where we were. For what? I don't want to see another needless loss."

I felt I had failed Dr. D in some way. How could I have been ignorant of his inner turmoil and yet claim I knew him well? Either I had been blind or lulled by his gregariousness. Or, like cancer, you can't see the inner menace unless it wants to be seen.

Dr. D and I had talked about Gabriel García Márquez's *Chronicle of a Death Foretold.* It's a favorite novel of mine because of its brevity and suspense, and its mystery and paradox about life's unavoidable misfortunes. A beautiful but poor girl, Ángela, is married to a wealthy man. But on the wedding night, he finds that she isn't a virgin, and he drags her back to her parents' home the same night. Who could have taken away her virginity? The bride, after her mother's merciless beatings, accuses, perhaps falsely, Santiago Nasar, a handsome, raffish, twenty-one-year-old man. Her twin brothers, close friends of Nasar, must kill him to restore the family's honor, and they express their intention brazenly to others. These are the telling points: it's a small town, and many know that Nasar is going to be killed, yet no one tries to stop the fatal event; and a friend who frantically searched for him to warn him couldn't find him in time. In the end, Nasar is fatally stabbed by the brothers at his own doorstep, with the knives they use to slaughter pigs.

Did Dr. D have any foretelling signs that had escaped me? It seemed that his life, in one respect, had paralleled *Chronicle*: we became urgently interested in him only after the violence had been committed.

And what about Alma? Alma means "soul." I had misjudged her, as I had her husband, because of her gentle soul, her appearance and manner. I had no idea that her soul could be so steely.

I came to admire Alma's courage, especially when I found out how she was treated after the funeral. Several of Dr. D's family members and friends—doctors among them—wouldn't forgive her. How could she desecrate his honor by airing his dirty laundry in public? But she bore the ostracism with dignity.

Why did the doctors have difficulty with Alma's bluntness? Was it because she forced us to look inside ourselves? Doctors have the highest suicide rate of any profession—every day, one doctor commits suicide in the US. This had hit home for me more than once. Three other colleagues in our community had killed themselves within a short time. The number of doctor suicides, regardless of gender—28 to 40 per 100,000—is more than twice that of the general population. Burnout and stress lead to depression, the prime culprit that instigates self-destruction. The main barrier to seeking treatment is the stigma attached to mental disorders.

Alma left a warning for me. With all the pain and anguish of my cancer patients I had to cope with, I became more watchful of *el diablo* than I was before.

"Death is the great equalizer," the sages say. The sages may be right on many things but not on this one.

Juan Garcia's funeral, too, revealed a few things that I was only vaguely aware of. He had been a faithful Catholic, then lapsed after his wife died. But he still wanted a church service. Catholic funeral rites can be long, but his was short. A lone wreath sat to one side of the casket, and about two dozen mourners attended. Juan's daughter from Houston silently wept. Her brother and I tried to comfort her, but it seemed she wanted to be left alone to grieve in her own way. I wondered if she faulted herself for not visiting her father. I came to know more about her from Juan in his final days. She had divorced her abusive husband and was struggling to raise three small children while working as a nurse's aide; at the same time, she was attending community college to become an LVN to improve her lot. We all have our personal handicaps that keep us from doing things despite our good intentions. But I have also seen how ill feeling, like a malignancy, has its own effect, and even a death doesn't change some hearts, be they family members or friends. Of course, this says something about the nature of these people as well. At least Juan's daughter had come to pay her last respects.

The young priest who was officiating tried to make the best out of the situation. He performed his obligatory prayers and recitations and talked obliquely of what I understood to be mercy and redemption. Finally, Alberto summarized the deceased's life. "My father wasn't an easy man to know, but he was a good, hardworking man. Then something snapped in him after my mother's death. He raised my sister and me the best way he knew. For that, I'm grateful."

Later, I learned from Alberto that Juan's funeral service became a bone of contention. Besides being a lapsed Catholic, as Alberto saw it, Juan had failed to give to the church's cause and coffer. This negligence raised a fundamental question among the church functionaries: "Does Juan deserve a formal church funeral?" Some were against extending this privilege, but the lenient hearts won. The priestly duties, however, were assigned to the junior-most cleric.

Juan's service was quite a contrast to the funeral of another doctor, whose wife was a socialite with influential connections. His elaborate memorial was held at his big church, which was full, and people who came late had to stand along the walls. The whole altar area was adorned with magnificent flowers. More revealing, the busy bishop himself, with his entourage, took time to lead the service. Seeing the pageantry reminded me of a Willa Cather story, *My Mortal Enemy*. In that story, John Driscoll was a rich benefactor of his church. When he died, no one had ever seen a funeral like his: "The bishop was there, and a flock of priests in gorgeous vestments. When the pallbearers arrived, Driscoll did not come to the church; the church came to him. The bishop and clergy went down the nave and met that great black coffin at the door..." And Driscoll himself entered the heavenly realm in grand style: "From the freshness of the roses and lilies, from the glory of the high altar, he had gone straight to the greater glory, through smoking censers and candles and stars."

Funeral prejudice, unfortunately, crosses religious and cultural boundaries. When I was a high school student, a famous professional drama company from Calcutta (now Kolkata) came to perform in our school town. All their actors and actresses were Hindus except one, who was a Muslim. In his performance, he had the role of a drunkard. In one scene, he vomited blood and collapsed. The audience thought it was a part of the drama, and they clapped and cheered. Only after the curtain was drawn did we discover that the man was dead. In real life, he happened to be an alcoholic, and it turned out that he had succumbed to bleeding esophageal varices, a grim complication of advanced cirrhosis of the liver.

A number of our mosque dignitaries wouldn't sanction a mosque funeral for him because, according to them, he had spent his life among the *beshyas* (prostitutes), meaning the accomplished actresses. A few of these opponents were outright hypocrites in the name of faith, for they had been admirers of the actor and had attended many of his shows. Once, they had openly extolled his virtues: "We're lucky to have a great artist like him in our town." But upon his death, he wasn't an artist anymore. The same people now said, "God punished him for his sinful life; that's why he died the way he did." We had a wise old imam who was tolerant: "The dead deserve compassion." He stood firm, and prevailed.

Through their deaths, as through their lives, my patients challenged me to examine my own self and assess what I had learned from my past and my present, what I had become and what I was yet to be.

EPILOGUE: EMPATHY MATTERS IN MEDICINE

A book of patients' stories cannot be complete without a story of a doctor who became a patient. Here is my own tale that compelled me to rethink practicing and nurturing empathy.

I used to think that as an active oncologist for thirty-five years, I was well versed on the subject. But I was wrong. It was only when, in a matter of seconds, I went from doctor to patient that I grasped its true significance.

I also came to understand the stark reality of being a patient. Susan Sontag said, "Everyone who is born holds dual citizenship, in the kingdom of the well and in the kingdom of the sick." Like my patients, I had left the realm of the well and had entered the realm of the sick.

A hiking trail that I had long taken for granted betrayed me one day. The stones on a steep path that appeared solid beneath my feet suddenly shifted, and I slipped hard, slid fast, and fell off a cliff. My right foot landed on a rock slab, crushing my right ankle badly, with five fractures.

I was taken to the emergency room of the hospital where I worked. My orthopedic colleague, Dr. K, took me to surgery. But as a result of the huge swelling of the joint from the trauma, he couldn't repair my ankle. He explained that cutting through the edematous muscles and tissues would impede healing and increase the chances of infection, which could turn nasty, compounding my problem. He was only able to temporarily stabilize my fractures. For this, he used an external fixator made of metal-alloy rods, which were drilled through my heel bone below and my shinbone above, and then fastened together by bolts and screws. He advised me that the definitive surgery should be done only after the swelling was gone. Meanwhile, I was in a lot of pain.

"The next operation won't be easy, though," he warned me, "so I'm referring you to Dr. B, a specialist in ankle orthopedics." Dr. B practiced in an academic center in a big city far from ours.

Seeing my alarmed expression, Dr. K softened his tone. "It's not pancreatic cancer, you know," he said. "You'll get better in time. Try to put up with the pain for a while."

I wasn't sure how to react to his words, words that were meant to comfort me. What he said was true—I was far luckier than any of my patients with pancreatic cancer. But that thought also brought on some unpleasant memories—how some of my pancreatic cancer patients had suffered. Would I suffer the same pain as those unfortunate souls, no matter how temporary? How capricious would my pain be? Doctors sometimes say things without thinking, and heaven knows how many times I have said similar things in my own practice.

Although it was arduous, I assiduously followed Dr. K's advice to reduce the edematous swelling of my joint and leg: diligent wound care and constant elevation of my foot on six pillows day and night. Diuretics are useless for traumatic and inflammatory edema, and it's hard to believe that even with all the advances in surgery, there's no high-tech cure for this kind of traumatic swelling. Only gravity slowly brings down the fluid accumulated in the muscles and tissues—hence, the old-fashioned remedy of elevation with pillows.

Even at home, I slept on a hospital bed. The metal hardware attached to my leg was painful and taxing. And night times sometimes turned into nightmares. If, during the oblivion of sleep, the fractured foot with the hardware slipped off the high pillows, I was wakened by piercing pain. So, I was restless most of the night, and that exhausted me to no end. I had access to codeine, a lower-tier narcotic, but it only made things worse for me. The pills dulled my brain and caused anorexia, nausea, and abdominal bloating. I could now see more clearly how much my cancer patients had to deal with besides their pain when I gave them narcotics.

I realized that my best chance for freedom was Dr. B, the ankle orthopedist I was referred to by Dr. K. Once my swelling subsided after about three weeks, I made the difficult trip to see him. I believed that he, being a fellow physician, would surely be empathetic to me and understand my suffering.

To my shock, my belief proved to be utterly misplaced. He was unfeeling and showed more interest in my fractures than in me. He seemed unaware that the joint was attached to a living being. He didn't bother to touch me and was aloof to the concerns I raised. I was just a technical challenge and nothing more.

"I've looked at your x-rays and scans," he said, "and you have a hell of a lot of fractures." He then scheduled my surgery. Desperate to get some personal attention, and unsure if he was aware of my profession, I told him that I was an oncologist. "That won't change your surgery," he said, and left.

After I settled into a hospital room, a young doctor came to my bedside. "I'm an orthopedic resident, assisting Dr. B today," he said.

He wanted to discuss one of my medications, an anticoagulant. "Why are you taking it?" he asked. "Did you have blood clots in the veins and lungs?" Then he was curt: "Have you stopped it? We can't do surgery if you haven't. We can't risk hemorrhage on the operating table."

I was glad he was being careful about my condition before the operation. I assured him that I didn't have blood clots and that my local orthopedist had given me the drug in the hope of preventing them. I also told him that I had stopped taking it before coming here, as I had been advised. Those were all the answers the young doctor was interested in, and he didn't ask me any more questions about my health. He, too, didn't even touch me. I could see that the young doctor was copying his mentor well. The orthopedic resident's only concern seemed to be the anticoagulant that was noted in my chart. Too much bleeding on the operating table would not only be bad for me but also for the surgeon's reputation. When the resident finished, a nurse gave me an injection. After that, I had no idea what had transpired until I woke up in the surgical recovery room. I was confused at first and wondered why I was in a strange place. Then I noticed a familiar face smiling at me—it was my wife, Jahanara (Ara).

"You've been in the recovery unit for six hours since the surgery, waiting to get a room on the floor," she said. "Surgery went fine." I reflexively looked at my right leg. It had a white cast, and the hardware was gone. I was relieved by the disappearance of those contraptions that had given me so much grief. Ara's presence and smile made me more alert—she had a way with me.

It dawned on me that Ara had been sitting by my side all throughout this ordeal, except when I was in the operating room. I felt a pang of guilt. This vivacious, beautiful woman who looked elegant in her saris looked haggard now. Her long, lush black hair was disheveled, and her eyes sunken, face dry. What had I done to her? Why did I go on that cursed hike when she asked me not to go to that hiking trail that day? Did she have some kind of premonition?

Finally, at midnight, I got a room on the surgical floor. By then, the analgesic effect of the anesthesia was gone, and I began to experience pain again. But this pain was of another kind, gnawing and oppressive. As the muscles and tissues of the operated ankle and leg progressively swelled again because of the cutting, they were compressed more and more by the hard cast surrounding them. This felt worse than when I had the hardware fixator, which at least provided room for the swelling to expand. I wanted badly to forestall the pain's increasing severity. I pressed the call button for the nurses to get an injection of morphine along with an antinausea medication.

"Someone made a mistake in keying in your narcotics," a nurse said. "I've called for a reorder."

Then there was more delay. "Only one pharmacist is on call at night," she said. "He's swamped, and narcotic injections have strict rules."

She didn't need to cite me the narcotic rules—I had lived with them during my long years of cancer practice. She was genuinely sorry and offered me an oral codeine combination. I was glad to accept it, but all it did was to make me more miserable with nausea and abdominal bloating, and it scarcely offered any pain relief. Soon I was overwhelmed with pain, and I felt like a condemned prisoner without hope. By the time the nurse finally gave me a morphine injection, it was about 4 a.m., four hours after my request.

Following the injection, I became peaceful and went to sleep. I wished I had stayed that way. But I was startled awake at 6 a.m. by Dr. B, who came to make his morning rounds. Without so much as saying "good morning," he held up an x-ray picture in front of me.

"Here's a copy of your x-ray after the surgery," he said, and then quickly described what he had done. "I've put in two plates and fourteen screws to align the bones, and some bone grafts to fill the gaps."

My eyes were blurry from the light, and I was still hazy from the morphine and exhaustion. I couldn't take it all in. (Only later, with Ara's compassionate help, could I understand what the doctor had said.)

After Dr. B finished with the x-ray, he grabbed his materials and hurried to leave the room. Holding the doorknob on his way out, he said, "You can go home this morning."

I didn't even have a chance to tell him about my ordeals at night. Ara, worried about my pain and debility, pleaded my case: "He's too sick to travel, Doctor, and we live far away from here."

Dr. B wasn't moved by her plea and barely paid attention to her. "He can rest in a hotel as good as he can in the hospital," he said. Then, as he walked off, he mentioned, "I'll check him in my office in two days. You can talk to the discharge planner."

I discovered that he had admitted me as an outpatient surgery, and I had already spent a night in the hospital. And he was a busy surgeon, and the hospital might lose money on me. One may see how unfair this discharge was and say that I had a right to complain about it. However, when you are ill, you are vulnerable, doctor or not. You sign all the forms the hospital puts in front of you because you have to, and this absolves the hospital of any questionable conduct. True, I didn't knowingly take part in any wrongdoing or condone it in my practice, but if I did, didn't my patients absolve me and my hospital by signing the consent forms?

I wish I could say that my experience is unique, but it is not. Countless patients can identify with me. Sadly, as I look back, I see that Dr. B's behavior was partly explained by the silence of our profession. After all, neither I, nor likely any other physician, ever reproached a colleague who fell far short on compassion and empathy.

Sure, advances in medicine are saving and improving the quality of our lives, as they did mine, and my own surgeon was technically skillful. And of course, technical knowledge and proficiency are essential in medicine. But by themselves, they do not ensure patients' welfare. For one important attribute, empathy, is an integral part of care. Empathy helps to build bonds between doctors and patients and lessens patients' anxiety and distress; in turn, it improves patient satisfaction and clinical outcome. I believe that physicians' empathy is particularly important for cancer patients, especially those who are on prolonged chemotherapy, since they see their oncologists so often, from weekly to monthly and so on, for years. It's easy to become dulled to their distress hearing the same complaints again and again.

A lack of empathy has another effect that's not obvious: a corrosive influence on the doctor's mindset. At least nine medical specialty groups have found that more than fifty procedures and tests currently performed by doctors have no demonstrable benefit, and they can even be harmful to patients. Although some tests and treatments are done with good intentions, others, unfortunately, are done for reasons that are less than altruistic. Surely, any empathetic physician would strive not to subject her or his patients to unnecessary tests or treatments. Moreover, a lack of empathy will also harm doctors' own interests: the public will become increasingly disenchanted with our profession, and then, over time, they will make greater demands on our practice—demands that are less empathetic to our difficulties and frustrations.

Sensitivity to others' anguish can't be taught through science alone. Though science is the basis of medicine, it can't grasp our life's trials, foibles, and incongruities. Empathy can be nurtured from the beginning of medical education. How? By teaching the humanities to medical students and trainees. Some medical schools take the issue more seriously than others. One of the former is the University of Texas Health Science Center in San Antonio, which advances the cause through its Charles E. Cheever Jr. Center for Medical Humanities & Ethics. (Disclosure: I serve on the advisory council of this center.)

"We recommit ourselves to the vision of preparing tomorrow's healers to act with compassion and justice . . . to bring ethics in action," said Ruth Berggren, MD, MACP, professor of medicine, and former director of the Cheever Center.

Ample stories in literature and the arts open our eyes to the subject. When I taught medical humanities to mostly premed students, I began with Anton Chekhov's classic short story "Ward No. 6" to draw their attention.

Dr. Andrei Yefimych is indifferent to the dehumanizing treatment of his patients. Then, by a quirk of fate, he becomes a patient in his own ward. Once the roles are reversed, he faces the same treatment his patients do. Chekhov, the doctor-writer, vividly describes the encounter between the new Yefimych and Nikita, a sadistic orderly in the ward. An excerpt follows (italics are mine):

Nikita quickly opened the door, rudely shoved Andrei Yefimych aside with his hands and knee, then swung and hit him in the face with his fist. Andrei Yefimych felt as if a huge salt wave had broken over him and was pulling him towards the bed; in fact, there was a salt taste in his mouth; his teeth were bleeding. He waved his arms as if trying to swim and got hold of someone's bed, and just then he felt Nikita hit him twice in the back.

Ivan Dmitrich [another patient in the ward] gave a loud cry. He, too, must have been beaten.

Then all was quiet. . . . Andrei Yefimych lay there with bated breath: he waited in terror to be hit again. It was as if someone had taken a sickle, plunged it into him, and twisted it several times in his chest and guts. He bit his pillow in pain and clenched his teeth, and suddenly, amidst the chaos, a dreadful, unbearable thought flashed clearly in his head, that *exactly the same pain must have been felt day after day, for years, by these people who now looked like black shadows in the moonlight. How could it happen that in the course of more than twenty years he had not known and had not wanted to know it?*

To be sure, this sort of flagrant violence is not practiced in modern hospitals, but we have our variations of it in subtler, insidious forms. The core point remains the same, so the story does serve a purpose. It leaves an impression on any medical student or trainee who is asked to contemplate the value of empathy, and on what would happen if the patient-doctor roles were reversed.

Poetry, too, has a way of enlightening us all. A poem can distill the essence of our feelings. Raymond Carver's poem "What the Doctor Said" tells about an encounter between a doctor and a patient with advanced cancer. Carver knew firsthand what it was to be a patient with a fatal disease. Like Chekhov, whom he admired and who coughed up blood because of tuberculosis of the lung, Carver coughed up blood because of cancer of the lung. He died of its metastasis to the brain and lungs at the age of fifty, in 1988. (Note: This poem doesn't have full punctuation.)

What the Doctor Said

He said it doesn't look good
he said it looks bad in fact real bad

he said I counted thirty-two of them on one lung before
I quit counting them
I said I'm glad I wouldn't want to know
about any more being there than that
he said are you a religious man do you kneel down
in forest groves and let yourself ask for help
when you come to a waterfall
mist blowing against your face and arms
do you stop and ask for understanding at those moments
I said not yet but I intend to start today
he said I'm real sorry he said
I wish I had some other kind of news to give you
I said Amen and he said something else
I didn't catch and not knowing what else to do
and not wanting him to have to repeat it
and me to have to fully digest it
I just looked at him
for a minute and he looked back it was then
I jumped up and shook hands with this man who'd just given me
something no one else on earth had ever given me
I may have even thanked him habit being so strong

Where else can you get such heartfelt, revealing exchanges between a doctor and a patient within such a brief space? While the doctor struggles to convey the diagnosis and its hopeless outcome and yet to be sympathetic, the patient struggles to absorb what the doctor says. It also tells of their distress, fear, and confusion, and about seeking solace from faith, mysticism, and nature. Moreover, we can visualize how the desperate patient is grasping for the last straw after the doomed news. You can't teach these things with science. In fact, the doctor knows the limits of science, which has no power to cure the terminal condition. That's why he doesn't ask the patient to turn to science for succor.

Along with literature, painting and other visual arts play a part in learning and teaching. If you pay attention to paintings and pictures on medicine and life, you notice things that you don't notice in pharmacology or physiology.

Also, we can't tutor and practice compassion and empathy unless we consider an integral part of health and healing: inequality in medicine, which affects all aspects of cancer care. Prostate cancer, for instance, is the commonest cancer in men and the second commonest cause of cancer death. Despite all the progress in its diagnosis and treatment, Black men are twice as likely to die of the disease and suffer more from its complications, like pain; bone metastasis with pain is frequent with this cancer. Unfortunately, there are racial disparities even in treating cancer pain. Black patients are less likely to receive an opioid prescription and often get lower doses compared to similar White patients. Here, another humanities field—music—comes to help. It has been documented that music therapy—patients' playing or listening to music—without drugs is effective in pain relief in both Black and White patients.

Music is universal, crossing race and culture. If it can at least equalize the quality of life by ameliorating pain—and music costs little or nothing—imparting its value to students is obvious.

I realize that while studying all the scientific complexities of medicine and dealing with the diversions of modern living, there's little time for anything else. But the complexity and diversions are all the more reason to save some room for arts and literature. Of course, any medical student or trainee can get certificates by learning only the science, but I have never forgotten my grandmother's admonition about education: it's more than earning certificates. Though unlettered, her lack of formal education was more than made up for by her incisive wisdom.

Years later, I was heartened to see a highly educated person, Arthur L. Horwich, a professor at the Yale School of Medicine, echo my grandmother's sentiment: "You may think you know a lot but there's really no substitute for realizing how little you know when facing a patient at the bedside."

We should instill into young doctors and would-be doctors that medicine is more of a calling than a profession. And a personal touch is a vital link between patients and doctors, even with the recent push for virtual practice since the COVID-19 crisis. A 2023 health survey in the US and five other affluent countries gave an insight into this: 77 percent of patients still prefer in-person connection with their medical practitioners to virtual ones. But there's another crucial link in this connection that's not talked about: medical school teachers. They must practice what they preach. I had been taught by many committed teachers in all the places I had been. Yet in more than a half a century as a student, trainee, practitioner, and sometimes a teacher, I have also seen the contrary type, who regurgitates textbooks and journals and gives short shrift to empathy and personal connection. This attitude breeds cynicism among learners and molds their thinking, which they will carry to their future careers.

Students and trainees do most of their bedside learning in hospitals. But many hospitals, too, are becoming more impersonal and uncaring, and it doesn't matter whether they are for-profit or nonprofit; both can be equally callous and cutthroat. Nonprofits get enormous tax breaks to provide care for the poorest people in their communities, and some nonprofits become wealthy at the expense of the taxpayers. In reality, nationwide nonprofits provide only about 2 percent of their expenses for charity care, and some wealthy ones even less than half of that. Hospitals must set examples to make medicine more patient-oriented, beyond earning money.

End-of-life care shouldn't be treated as the stepchild of medicine. Physicians and students need to believe that caring for the dying is as noble as caring for others. And the quality of life of the dying is just as important. Communicating with terminal patients and talking about death is difficult for young minds, but this can be overcome if we instruct them in a measured tone.

In my student and postgraduate years in Dhaka, New York, and Houston, the overriding concern was teaching how to cure and save lives, and teaching about end-of-life was an afterthought or avoided altogether. Things have progressed since then, but we still have a long way to go. This is especially pertinent because medical technology is advancing faster than before, and we can keep the terminally ill elderly alive in the ICU longer and longer, to their detriment. I have seen enough thoughtless CPRs inflicted on them, traumatizing their last days before their death. The uncomfortable fact is that the fastest growing population is the oldest old, eighty-five years and above, and with that, there will be more afflictions and prolonged debility for many. We will then be forced to confront more gray areas in medicine, and our compassion and empathy will be tested. We have no choice but to learn and teach how to deal with this newer world.

ACKNOWLEDGMENTS

W riting is hard work for me as for many other writers, but Travis Snyder made it easier with his invaluable advice and keen insight. Thank you so much, Travis, for being my editor and taking personal interest in the book. Senior editor Christie Perlmutter has used her unusual talent and patience to improve the manuscript, as has senior designer Hannah Gaskamp; I can't thank them enough. Also, many thanks to copy editor Carly Kahl and marketing manager John Brock for their help.

I appreciate Sarah Russo's and Gene Taft's help to reach a wider audience for the book. Thank you, Sarah, for being such a sympathetic teacher.

I am indebted to two of the most distinguished experts in the cancer field, both from MD Anderson Cancer Center: Gabriel Hortobagyi, chair emeritus of the Department of Breast Medical Oncology, for reviewing the breast cancer story in part 2; and Hagop Kantarjian, chair of the Department of Leukemia, for reviewing the leukemia and myeloma stories in parts 1 and 3. Any mistakes, however, are all mine.

The chapter "Empathy Matters" was published in *The Oncologist* in 2014 in a different form.

Thanks to Jonathan Balcombe, an accomplished writer on the natural world, for his suggestions; and Yasmin von Dassow, a talented marine biologist and a discerning reader and editor, for her help in many ways, in particular, with the references. And I appreciate my agent, Elizabeth (Liz) Trupin-Pulli, for her advice; Tom Brady for his help with my technical problems; Lisa Bradley at the Texas Tech University Museum Publications for suggesting Travis Snyder.

I am deeply grateful to all my patients for sharing their lives with me and trusting me in their trying times of cancer treatments. They taught and inspired me a great deal, and I hope the readers, including those in medicine, will gain from their experiences. The identities of the patients here have been concealed, and any resemblance to anyone would be a coincidence. I should note that though the daily basic hurdles of cancer patients and their oncologists remain the same, diagnoses, treatments, and prognoses are advancing for the better.

With increasing involvement of many intermediaries between doctors and patients in medical care, it's often forgotten that nurses are the unsung heroes of medicine. They seem to be remembered by the hospital administrators only when a wing or two of a hospital has to be closed because of their shortage. I have been fortunate to work with many dedicated nurses, and I owe thanks to many in the profession, but due to lack of space, I mention only the following because of my long years with them in my cancer practice: the late Eileen Ann Strickland (the first oncology-certified nurse in West Texas), Dorethea Jackson DeWitt, Michelle Gerhart, Debbie Harris, Lea Henderson, Pam Kuhlmey, Melanie Thomas, Irene Watson, Ruby Wilson, and Mike Wood.

My practicing career began with the West Texas Medical Associates (WTMA), a first-rate, patient-oriented, multi-specialty group, formed by colleagues and me in 1976, under the leadership of the late Jack Rice and Sterling Gillis. WTMA was socially conscious as well and founded the WTMA Distinguished Lectureship in Science Honoring Dr. Roy Moon—commonly known as the Moon Lecture—which my colleagues and I financed and advanced for forty-five years since 1977, to promote science education and research to the students and the public. It's a joint program with Angelo State University (ASU), and it brings world-class scientists to the campus annually to fulfill that cause. The lecturers have included fifteen Nobel Laureates and giants in science such as Linus Pauling, Har Gobind Khorana, Kip Thorne, Ahmed Zewail, Mary-Claire King, Lynn Margulis, and Huda Zoghbi. The lectureship was the brainchild of the late Dr. Ralph Chase to memorialize our revered colleague Roy Moon, both of whom were my mentors. WTMA's recent demise because of the COVID-19 pandemic and other intractable forces beyond its control is an unfortunate chapter in San Angelo medicine, as is the loss of the independent San Angelo Community Medical Center, once the primary hospital for my patients.

ASU has been a part of my career in one form or another since 1975, and the Moon Lecture has been a success due to its selection committee members from the ASU science faculty and WTMA doctors, led by the deans of sciences as chairs, and the wide participation of the students and the public. I have enjoyed the friendship and support of the ASU deans and professors, including Paul Sweats, dean of the College of Science and Engineering and the current chair of the Moon selection committee; my Department of Biology faculty colleagues, among whom are Loren Ammerman, who kindly directed me to the Texas Tech University Press, Michael Dixon, Laurel Fohn, Nick Negovetich, Ben Skipper, and Russell Wilke. I also appreciate the friendship of many of the current and former faculty members of the Department of English and Modern Languages: Karen Cody, Ewa Davis, Chris Ellery, Mary Ellen Hartje, Erin Ashworth-King, and Laurence Musgrove. Along with other colleagues, they spearheaded the annual ASU Writers Conference in Honor of Elmer Kelton, who also influenced me.

I thank my former WTMA colleagues who are still in practice—Hector Acton, Ross Alexander, Robert Alexander, Warren Conway, Ted Hackl, Deborah Hajovsky, and Darrell Herrington—for maintaining their friendship and courtesy to Jahanara (Ara) and me and our family despite the drastic changes in the current medical scene.

It's been a privilege to serve as an advisory council member of the Charles E. Cheever Jr. Center for Medical Humanities and Ethics at the University of Texas Health Science Center in San Antonio. For many years, my association with Ruth Berggren, Francisco and Graciela Cigarroa, Marvin Forland, Mary Henrich, Jason Morrow, Rachel Pearson, Jerald Winakur, and other council and faculty members have broadened my horizons in medical humanities and ethics.

I have also been privileged to be a part of higher education as a trustee—now a senior trustee—of Austin College in Sherman, Texas, an excellent liberal arts college, which does more than its share to mold young minds to better the country and the planet. I appreciate the friendship of Oscar Page and Marjorie Hass, its former presidents; Steven O'Day, the current president; and my former trustee colleagues, a few of whom are: Robert M. Johnson, a former Board of Trustees chair, Susan Cuellar, Jacqueline Cooper, Rebecca Gafford, Mary Ann Harris, Sharon King, Becky Sykes, Todd Williams, and Mike Wright; the Austin College faculty members, especially Henry Bucher, a longtime Humanities faculty scholar; and the Austin College staff, in particular Genna Bethel, Gillian Locke, and Heidi Rushing. Austin College's Posey Leadership Award (ACPLA) gives annual recognition to a servant leader who has changed people's lives for the better. I have been enlightened by being on its selection committee, and I thank all the members for sharing their ideas and thoughts with me: among others, Bob Mong, current president of the University of North Texas at Dallas and a former editor in chief of the *Dallas Morning News*, who had given me pages for many of my pieces for a long time, and whose numerous awards include one that is of immediate relevance to this book, the National Empathy Award; the current ACPLA Committee Chair Brent Christopher, former Chairs Jim Moroney and Stan Woodward; and Tim Smith, president of the Posey Family Foundation.

I am particularly thankful to several friends for their sustained generosity: Jerald Winakur, physician, memoirist, essayist, and poet, whose wisdom and encouragement have kept me going during my dry periods of writing; Clare and Jack Ratliff; Dr. Alessandra Ferrajoli at the MD Anderson leukemia faculty for being a caring physician for two decades for one of my dearest family members; and John Cargile.

My children and my immediate family members come to my aid in times of need, and I thank them all: Anowar, Ayub, Gulshan, Happy, Mickey, Niva, Prince, Sean, and Yasmin. One young couple deserves special mention: Ataur and Mily Rahman, who have gone beyond the call of duty to stand by my side when I need immediate help. And the newer generations, including Jason, Haseeb, and Ryan give me hope for a better world.

Above all, I owe an everlasting debt to one soul, my wife and my life partner, Jahanara (Ara), whose unending love and sustenance have anchored me throughout our trials and travails.

REFERENCES AND SUGGESTED READINGS

INTRODUCTION
Novel treatment for Hodgkin's disease:
DeVita, V. T., A. A. Serpick, and P. P. Carbone. "Combination Chemotherapy in the Treatment of Advanced Hodgkin's Disease." *Annals of Internal Medicine* 73 (1970): 881–95. doi: https://doi.org/10.7326/0003-4819-73-6-881.

CHAPTER 1
Overview of multiple myeloma and breast cancer from National Cancer Institute:
National Cancer Institute. "Breast Cancer—Patient Version." https://www.cancer.gov/types/breast.
National Cancer Institute. "Plasma Cell Neoplasms (Including Multiple Myeloma)—Patient Version." https://www.cancer.gov/types/myeloma.
From Mayo Clinic:
Mayo Clinic. "Breast Cancer." https://www.mayoclinic.org/diseases-conditions/breast-cancer/symptoms-causes/syc-20352470.
Mayo Clinic. "Multiple Myeloma." https://www.mayoclinic.org/diseases-conditions/multiple-myeloma/symptoms-causes/syc-20353378.
Overview of antibiotic resistance:
Levy, S. B. "The Challenge of Antibiotic Resistance." *Scientific American* 278, no. 3 (1998): 46–53.
Story of the cell:
Mukherjee, S. *The Song of the Cell: An Exploration of Medicine and the New*

Human. New York: Scribner, 2022.

CHAPTER 2

Novel use of dexamethasone in myeloma treatment:

Alexanian, R., M. A. Dimopoulos, K. Delasalle, and B. Barlogie. "Primary Dexamethasone Treatment of Multiple Myeloma." *Blood* 80, no. 4 (1992): 887–90.

Overview of hospice care and palliative care from the National Institute on Aging:

National Institute on Aging. "What Are Palliative Care and Hospice Care?" https://www.nia.nih.gov/health/what-are-palliative-care-and-hospice-care#hospice.

From the American Cancer Society:

American Cancer Society. "What Is Hospice Care?" https://www.cancer.org/treatment/end-of-life-care/hospice-care/what-is-hospice-care.html.

Improvement of patient and family experience by hospice:

Kumar, P., A. A. Wright, L. A. Hatfield, J. S. Temel, and N. L. Keating. "Family Perspectives on Hospice Care Experiences of Patients with Cancer." *Journal of Clinical Oncology* 35, no. 4 (2017): 432.

Shockney, L. D. "How to Help Terminally Ill Patients Find Peace in the Dying Process." *The ASCO Post,* October 10, 2019, 92–93. https://ascopost.com/issues/october-10-2019/how-to-help-terminally-ill-patients-find-peace-in-the-dying-process/.

Wallston, K., C. Burger, R. Smith, and R. Baugher. "Comparing the Quality of Death for Hospice and Non-hospice Cancer Patients." *Medical Care* 26, no. 2 (1988): 177–82.

Problems with the for-profit hospice system:

Whoriskey, P. and D. Keating. "Hospice Firms Draining Billions from Medicare." *The Washington Post*, December 26, 2013. https://www.washingtonpost.com/business/economy/medicare-rules-create-a-booming-business-in-hospice-care-for-people-who-arent-dying/2013/12/26/4ff75bbe-68c9-11e3-ae56-22de072140a2_story.html.

CHAPTER 3

On narcotics for cancer patients:

Rahman, F. "Narcotics for Cancer Patients." *The New York Times*, June 12, 1987, A31. https://www.nytimes.com/1987/06/12/opinion/narcotics-for-cancer-patients.html.

A bioethicist on pain:

Rieder, T. N. "The Painful Truth About Pain." *Nature* 573 (2019): S16–S16.2.

Understanding chronic pain and its multidisciplinary management:

Darbha, V., L. King, and A. Westbrook. "They Live in Constant Pain, but Their Doctors Won't Help Them." *New York Times*, August 17, 2023. https://www.nytimes.com/2023/08/17/opinion/opioids-chronic-pain-patients.html. A short video about the firsthand accounts of patients who are victims of chronic severe pain and their doctors' refusal to prescribe opioids. It is worth watching to understand the current pathetic scene in pain control.

Odling-Smee, L. "Chronic Pain: The Long Road to Discovery." *Nature* 615 (2023): 782–86.

"Treat Pain as a Priority, Not an Afterthought." Editorial. *Nature* 615 (2023): 765.

Author's advocacy for hospice programs:

Rahman, F. "An Alternative to Kevorkian's Prescription." *Wall Street Journal*, November 2, 1995.

CHAPTER 4

Report of breast cancer study fraud:

Maugh, T. H., II, and R. Mestel. "Key Breast Cancer Study was a Fraud." *The Los Angeles Times*, April 27, 2001. https://www.latimes.com/archives/la-xpm-2001-apr-27-mn-56336-story.html.

Original fraudulent study:

Bezwoda, W. R., L. Seymour, and R. D. Dansey. "High-dose Chemotherapy with Hematopoietic Rescue as Primary Treatment for Metastatic Breast Cancer: A Randomized Trial." *Journal of Clinical Oncology* 13, no. 10 (1995): 2483–89.

Retraction of the fraudulent study:

"Retraction for Bezwoda." *Journal of Clinical Oncology* 19, no. 11 (2001): 2973. doi: 10.1200/JCO.2001.19.11.2973.

High cost of Revlimid:

Kodjak, A. "How a Drugmaker Gamed the System to Keep Generic Competition Away." *Shots: Health News from NPR*. National Public Radio, May 2018. https://www.npr.org/sections/health-shots/2018/05/17/571986468/how-a-drugmaker-gamed-the-system-to-keep-generic-competition-away.

On research funding by the public:

Rahman, F. "The Public's Share of Medical Research." *The New York Times,* April 26, 1992, F13. https://www.nytimes.com/1992/04/26/business/forum-the-publics-share-of-medical-research.html.

Comments from patients and others on author's oncology practice and retirement:

Morris, D. "Local Oncologist Retires with Love and Respect After 35 Years." *The San Angelo Standard-Times,* July 4, 2011. http://archive.gosanangelo.com/news/local-oncologist-retires-with-love-and-respect-after-35-years-ep-439776892-356733091.html/.

Author's *Harvard Review* reference:

Rahman, F. "My Brother the Imam: Metamorphosis of a Novelist." *Harvard Review* 8 (1995): 122–25.

Author's *Lancet* memoir excerpts:

Rahman F. "Amulets and Poems: One Healer's Beginnings." *The Lancet* 350 (1997): 1848–49.

Rahman F. "Angels and Spirits in the World of Illness." *The Lancet* 352 (1998): 1218–19.

The story of bone marrow transplant:

Appelbaum, F. *Living Medicine: Don Thomas, Marrow Transplantation, and Cell Therapy Revolution.* Rochester, MN: Mayo Clinic Press, 2023.

Hubris in cancer medicine:

Raza, A. *The First Cell and the Human Costs of Pursuing Cancer to the Last.* New York: Basic Books, 2020.

CHAPTER 5

Rachel Carson's surgeon lied to her about her breast cancer diagnosis:

Groopman, Jerome. "The Sexual Politics of Cancer." *The New York Times,* January 9, 2000. https://www.nytimes.com/2000/01/09/books/ the-sexual-politics-of-cancer.html.

A history of surgical chauvinism and sexual politics in breast cancer:

Leopold, E. *A Darker Ribbon: Breast Cancer, Women, and the Doctors in the Twentieth Century.* Boston: Beacon Press, 2000.

Surgery may not be needed for some breast cancer patients:

The University of Texas MD Anderson Cancer Center. "Breast Biopsies After Neoadjuvant Chemotherapy Accurately Predict Presence of Residual Breast Cancer." News release. December 2019. https://www. mdanderson.org/newsroom/breast-biopsies-after-neoadjuyant-chemo- therapy-accurately-predict-presence-of-residual-breast-cancer.h00- 159308568.html.

The role of gut microbes in health and disease: a supplemental issue with multiple articles by multiple authors:

Brody, H., ed. "The Gut Microbe: Exploring the Microbes that Affect Human Health." *Nature* 577 (2020): S1-25.

CHAPTER 6

Hormone receptors in breast cancer:

Yip, C. H., and A. Rhodes. "Estrogen and Progesterone Receptors in Breast Cancer." *Future Oncology* 10, no. 14 (2014): 2293–301.

Thromboembolism with Tamoxifen use:

Hernandez, R. K., H. T. Sørensen, L. Pedersen, J. Jacobsen, and T. L. Lash. "Tamoxifen Treatment and Risk of Deep Venous Thrombosis and Pulmonary Embolism: A Danish Population-based Cohort Study." *Cancer* 115, no. 19 (2009): 4442–49. doi: 10.1002/cncr.24508.

WHO: Breast cancer is the commonest cancer in the world:

Arnold, M., E. Morgan, H. Rumgay, A. Mafra, D. Singh, M. Laversanne, et al. "Current and Future Burden of Breast Cancer: Global Statistics for 2020 and 2040." *Breast*, September 2, 2022. https://doi.org/10.1016/j. breast.2022.08.010.

CHAPTER 8

Current thinking of different organizations on mammogram guidelines:

Centers for Disease Control. "Screening for Breast Cancer." https://
www.cdc.gov/breast-cancer/screening/index.html#:~:text=Breast%20
cancer%20screening%20can%20help,a%20mammogram%20every%20
2%20years.

CHAPTER 9

Cardiotoxicity of 5-fluorouracil:

Polk, A., K. Vistisen, M. Vaage-Nilsen, and D. L. Nielsen. "A Systematic Review of the Pathophysiology of 5-fluorouracil-induced Cardiotoxicity." *BMC Pharmacology and Toxicology* 15 (2014): 47. doi: https://doi. org/10.1186/2050-6511-15-47.

Cardiotoxicity of Doxorubicin:

Chatterjee, K., J. Zhang, N. Honbo, and J. S. Karliner. "Doxorubicin Cardiomyopathy." *Cardiology* 115, no. 2 (2010): 155–62. doi: https:// doi.org/10.1159/000265166.

Flawed and fraudulent clinical studies:

Else, H. "Papers Co-authored by Nobel Laureate Raise Concerns." *Nature* 611 (2022): 19–20.

Noorden, R. V. "How Many Clinical Trials Can't be Trusted?" *Nature* 619 (2023): 455–58.

CHAPTER 10

Life of Ayub Khan Ommaya of the Ommaya reservoir:

Watts, G. "Ayub Khan Ommaya." *The Lancet* 372, no. 9649 (2008): 1540. doi: https://doi.org/10.1016/S0140-6736(08)61642-6.

The place of belief or unbelief in the face of loss and suffering:

Rahman, F. "A Doctor's Journey to the World of Faith." *Tex Med* 91 (1995):12, 29–30.

Symposium presentation in Corina Johnson's story:

Rahman, F. "Adriamycin and Velban Infusion for Breast Cancer in Advanced Age." Presented at the 8th Annual San Antonio Breast

Cancer Symposium. November 7–8, 1985.

Rahman, F. "Adriamycin and Velban Infusion for Breast Cancer in Advanced Age." *Proceedings of the American Society of Clinical Oncology* 4: 55.

No surgery for selected early breast cancer:

Kuerer, H. M., B. D. Smith, S. Krishnamurthy, et al. "Eliminating Breast Surgery for Invasive Breast Cancer in Exceptional Responders to Neoadjuvant Systemic Therapy: A Multicenter Phase 2 Trial." *Lancet Oncology* 23 (2022):1517–24.

Women suffering from disabling radical mastectomy:

Mukherjee, S. *The Laws of Medicine: Field Notes from an Uncertain Science.* TED Books. New York: Simon & Schuster, 2015, 59–61.

CHAPTER 11

Overview of leukemia from the National Cancer Institute:

National Cancer Institute. "Leukemia—Patient Version." https://www.cancer.gov/types/leukemia.

From the Mayo Clinic:

Mayo Clinic. "Chronic Myelogenous Leukemia." https://www.mayoclinic.org/diseases-conditions/chronic-myelogenous-leukemia/symptoms-causes/syc-20352417.

Philadelphia chromosome discovery:

Nowell, P., and D. Hungerford. "A Minute Chromosome in Human Chronic Granulocytic Leukemia." *Science* 132 (1960): 1497.

Cover story on Interferon:

"Interferon: The IF Drug for Cancer." *Time*, March 31, 1980.

FDA approval of alpha-interferon (Otis Bowen quote):

Fram, A. "Government Allows First Prescription use of Cancer Drug." *AP News*, June 4, 1986. https://apnews.com/fc9cdfd08bbdcb9923046cd799d9d6ca.

Discovery and use of Imatinib:

Deininger, M., E. Buchdunger, and B. J. Druker. "The Development of Imatinib as a Therapeutic Agent for Chronic Myeloid Leukemia." *Blood* 105, no. 7 (2005): 2640–53. doi: https://doi.org/10.1182/blood-2004-08-3097.

Kantarjian, H., S. O'Brien, E. Jabbour, et al. "Improved Survival in Chronic Myeloid Leukemia Since Introduction of Imatinib: A Single-institution Historical Experience." *Blood* 119, no. 9 (March 1, 2012). doi:10.1182/blood-2011-08-358135.

Kantarjian, H., C. Sawyers, A. Hochhaus, F. Guilhot, C. Schiffer, C. Gambacorti-Passerini, D. Niederwieser, D. Resta, R. Capdeville, U. Zoellner, and M. Talpaz. "Hematologic and Cytogenetic Responses to Imatinib Mesylate in Chronic Myelogenous Leukemia." *New England Journal of Medicine* 346, no. 9 (2002): 645–52.

National Cancer Institute. "How Imatinib Transformed Leukemia Treatment and Cancer Research." April 11, 2018. https://www.cancer.gov/research/progress/discovery/Gleevec.

CHAPTER 12

High cost of Gleevec:

Drugs.com. "Gleevec Prices, Coupons and Patient Assistance Programs." Accessed March 2020. https://www.drugs.com/price-guide/gleevec.

Kantarjian, H. "The Arrival of Generic Imatinib into the U.S. Market: An Educational Event." *The ASCO Post*, May 25, 2016. https://ascopost.com/issues/may-25-2016/the-arrival-of-generic-imatinib-in-to-the-us-market-an-educational-event/.

Cost of Zofran:

Drugs.com. "Zofran ODT Prices, Coupons and Patient Assistance Programs." Accessed March 2020. https://www.drugs.com/price-guide/zofran-odt.

US taxpayers' funding of drug research and development versus exorbitant costs of drugs:

Rahman, F. "The Public's Share of Medical Research." *The New York Times*, April 26, 1992, section 3, 13. https://www.nytimes.com/1992/04/26/business/forum-the-publics-share-of-medical-research.html.

Kantarjian quote:

Kantarjian, H. Interview by Lesley Stahl. *60 Minutes*, October 5, 2014. Transcript. https://www.cbsnews.com/news/the-cost-of-cancer-drugs/.

Forbes opinion piece on the _60 Minutes_ episode:

Herper, Matthew. "'60 Minutes' Just Attacked High Drug Prices. Here's What You Should Know." _Forbes_, October 5, 2014. https://www.forbes. com/sites/matthewherper/2014/10/05/60-minutes-just-attacked-high-drug-prices-heres-what-you-should-know/#30901969839a.

Doctors' perspectives on high-cost cancer drugs:

Experts in Chronic Myeloid Leukemia. "The Price of Drugs for Chronic Myeloid Leukemia (CML) is a Reflection of the Unsustainable Prices of Cancer Drugs: From the Perspective of a Large Group of CML Experts." _Blood_ 121, no. 22 (2013): 4439–42. doi: https://doi. org/10.1182/blood-2013-03-490003.

Kantarjian, H., D. Steensma, J. R. Sanjuan, A. Elshaug, and D. Light. "High Cancer Drug Prices in the United States: Reasons and Proposed Solutions." _Journal of Oncology Practice_ 10, no. 4 (2014): e208–e211.

Crippling financial toxicity of cancer:

Collado, L., and I. Brownell. "The Crippling Financial Toxicity of Cancer in the United States." _Cancer Biology & Therapy_ 20 (2019):1301–03.

Lewis, K., as told to Jo Cavallo. "Overcoming Financial Toxicity from Cancer." _The ASCO Post_, August 10, 2023. https://ascopost.com/ issues/august-10-2023/overcoming-financial-toxicity-from-cancer/.

CHAPTER 13

Larson regimen:

Larson, R. A., R. K. Dodge, C. P. Burns, E. J. Lee, R. M. Stone, P. Schulman, D. Duggan, F. R. Davey, R. E. Sobol, and S. R. Frankel. "A Five-drug Remission Induction Regimen with Intensive Consolidation for Adults with Acute Lymphoblastic Leukemia: Cancer and Leukemia Group B Study 8811." _Blood_ 85, no. 8 (1995): 2025–37. doi:https://doi.org/10.1182/blood.V85.8.2025.bloodjournal8582025.

In death and disease—and in an epidemic—how some are caring and some are self-serving; the story mimics today's COVID-19 pandemic and how it's exposing our true character:

Camus, A. _The Plague_. Everyman's Library. New York: Knopf, 2004.

Rahman, F. "COVID-19 and My Days Among Cholera and Smallpox." _San Angelo Standard-Times_, May 30, 2020.

CHAPTER 14
Nilotinib use:

Kantarjian, H., F. Giles, L. Wunderle, K. Bhalla, S. O'Brien, B. Wassmann, C. Tanaka, P. Manley, P. Rae, W. Mietlowski, and K. Bochinski. "Nilotinib in Imatinib-resistant CML and Philadelphia Chromosome–positive ALL." *New England Journal of Medicine* 354, no. 24 (2006): 2542–51.

CHAPTER 16
Overview of ovarian cancer from the National Cancer Institute:

National Cancer Institute. "Ovarian, Fallopian Tube, and Primary Peritoneal Cancer—Patient Version." https://www.cancer.gov/types/ovarian.

From the Mayo Clinic:

Mayo Clinic. "Ovarian Cancer." https://www.mayoclinic.org/diseases-conditions/ovarian-cancer/symptoms-causes/syc-20375941.

Cancer statistics in the oldest old:

American Cancer Society. "2019 Special Section: Cancer in the Oldest Old." *Cancer Facts and Figures 2019*. 2019. https://www.cancer.org/content/dam/cancer-org/research/cancer-facts-and-statistics/annual-cancer-facts-and-figures/2019/cancer-facts-and-figures-special-section-cancer-in-the-oldest-old-2019.pdf.

Author's article on Medicare and elder care:

Rahman, F. "Medicare Makes a Wrong Diagnosis." *The New York Times*, January 23, 1986, A27. https://www.nytimes.com/1986/01/23/opinion/medicare-makes-a-wrong-diagnosis.html.

Conflict between Taxol production and yew tree preservation:

Kolata, G. "Tree Yields a Cancer Treatment, but Ecological Cost May be High." *The New York Times*, May 13, 1991, A1. https://www.nytimes.com/1991/05/13/us/tree-yields-a-cancer-treatment-but-ecological-cost-may-be-high.html.

Life of Michael E. DeBakey, and his life-and-death surgery at the age of ninety-seven:

Altman, L. K. "The Man on the Table Devised the Surgery." *The New York Times*, December 25, 2006.

Oransky, I. "Michael E. DeBakey." *The Lancet* 372, no. 9638 (2008): 530. doi: https://doi.org/10.1016/S0140-6736(08)61223-4.

Winters, W. L. *Houston Hearts: A History of Cardiovascular Surgery and Medicine and the Methodist DeBakey Heart and Vascular Center at Houston Methodist Hospital.* Elisha Freeman Publishing, 2014.

CHAPTER 17

Symposium presentation based on patient with B12 deficiency:

Rahman, F. "Pernicious Anemia with Neuropsychiatric Disorders and Normal Bone Marrow." Presentation at the American Federation for Clinical Research, New York City. *Clinical Research* 37, no. 3 (September 23, 1989): 854A.

CHAPTER 18

Wordsworth poem:

Wordsworth, W. "Ode: Intimations of Immortality from Recollections of Early Childhood." 1804. https://www.poetryfoundation.org/poems/45536/ode-intimations-of-immortality-from-recollections-of-early-childhood.

Terrible suffering of the people of West Texas from a severe, protracted drought:

Kelton, Elmer. *The Time It Never Rained.* Fort Worth: TCU Press, 1984.

CHAPTER 19

Overview of hepatocellular carcinoma (liver cancer) from the National Cancer Institute:

National Cancer Institute. "Liver and Bile Duct Cancer." https://www.cancer.gov/types/liver.

From the Mayo Clinic:

Mayo Clinic. "Liver Cancer." https://www.mayoclinic.org/diseases-conditions/liver-cancer/symptoms-causes/syc-20353659.

Rural veterans' lack of access to VA care:

Lawrence, Q. "A Benefit for Rural Vets: Getting Health Care Close to

Home." *Morning Edition*, National Public Radio, October 13, 2014.
https://www.npr.org/sections/health-shots/2014/10/13/354307706/a-benefit-for-rural-vets-getting-health-care-close-to-home.

Hepatocellular carcinoma statistics and mortality rates:

National Cancer Institute. "Surveillance, Epidemiology, and End Results
Program." https://seer.cancer.gov/statfacts/.

Hepatitis C rates in the United States:

Centers for Disease Control and Prevention. "Hepatitis C." https://www.
cdc.gov/hepatitis/hcv/index.htm.

Hepatitis B rates in the United States:

Centers for Disease Control and Prevention. "Hepatitis B." https://www.
cdc.gov/hepatitis/hbv/index.htm.

Connection between hepatitis B and opioid abuse:

Harris, A. M., K. Iqbal, S. Schillie, J. Britton, M. A. Kainer, S. Tressler,
and C. Vellozzi. "Increases in Acute Hepatitis B Virus Infections—
Kentucky, Tennessee, and West Virginia, 2006–2013." *Morbidity
and Mortality Weekly Report* 65 (2016): 47–50. doi: http://dx.doi.
org/10.15585/mmwr.mm6503a2external icon.

Worldwide hepatitis C and B rates:

Nuila, R. *The People's Hospital: Hope and Peril in American Medicine.*
New York: Scribner, 2023.

World Health Organization. "Hepatitis B Fact Sheet." 2019. https://www.
who.int/news-room/fact-sheets/detail/hepatitis-b.

World Health Organization. "Hepatitis C Fact Sheet." 2019. https://www.
who.int/news-room/fact-sheets/detail/hepatitis-c.

CHAPTER 20

Nexavar cost in the US:

Drugs.com. "Nexavar Prices, Coupons and Patient Assistance Programs."
Accessed March 2020. https://www.drugs.com/price-guide/nexavar.

Nexavar cost in Canada:

Committee to Evaluate Drugs, Ontario Ministry of Health and Long-Term
Care. "Sorafenib (for Hepatocellular Carcinoma)." 2009. http://www.
health.gov.on.ca/en/pro/programs/drugs/ced/pdf/nexavar.pdf.

Average out-of-pocket cost percentage and Kantarjian quote:

Kantarjian, H. "Will the Trump Administration's Plan to Reduce Cancer Drug Prices Work?" *The ASCO Post*, December 25, 2018. https://www. ascopost.com/issues/december-25-2018/will-the-trump-administration-s-plan-to-reduce-cancer-drug-prices-work/.

Dyson quote:

Dyson, J., as told to J. Cavallo. "Cancer Has Given Me the Life I Was Meant to Live." *The ASCO Post*, February 25, 2019. https://www. ascopost.com/issues/february-25-2019/cancer-has-given-me-the-life-i-was-meant-to-live/.

Bias against minorities in cancer care:

Cavallo, Jo. "Is Implicit Bias Contributing to Time Disparities in Goals-of-care Conversations with Minority Patients? A Conversation with Cardinale B. Smith, MD, PhD." *The ASCO Post*, October 10, 2019, 1, 13–15. https://ascopost.com/news/september-2019/is-implicit-bias-contributing-to-time-disparities-in-conversations-with-minority-pa/.

Doctor-patient communication can't be replaced by a computer screen:

Holland, J. C., and J. F. Holland. "The More Things Change, the More They Stay the Same." *The ASCO Post*, July 10, 2014, 1, 34. https://ascopost.com/issues/july-10-2014/the-more-things-change-the-more-they-stay-the-same/.

Medicine as an art, from a top leader in the cancer field:

Simone, J. V. "The Practice of Medicine Is an Art." *Oncology Times* 35, no. 9 (2013): 12.

CHAPTER 21

Lack of prestige and compensation deters doctors from family medicine:

Mitra, A. "Why Don't Young Doctors Want to Work in Primary Care?" *The Pulse*, WHYY Radio/National Public Radio, June 23, 2016. https://whyy.org/segments/why-dont-young-doctors-want-to-work-in-primary-care/.

Number of US inpatient surgeries, 2010:

Centers for Disease Control and Prevention, National Center for

Health Statistics. "National Hospital Discharge Survey: 2010; Table, Procedures by Selected Patient Characteristics—Number by Procedure Category and Age." Atlanta: CDC, 2010. http://www.cdc.gov/nchs/nhds/nhds_tables.htm.

High rate of medical overtreatment in the US:

Lyu, H., T. Xu, D. Brotman, B. Mayer-Blackwell, M. Cooper, M. Daniel, E. C. Wick, V. Saini, S. Brownlee, and M. A. Makary. "Overtreatment in the United States." *PloS One* 12, no. 9 (2017): e0181970. doi: https://doi.org/10.1371/journal.pone.0181970.

Overuse of heart implants:

Al-Khatib, S. M., A. Hellkamp, J. Curtis, D. Mark, E. Peterson, G. D. Sanders, P. A. Heidenreich, A. F. Hernandez, L. H. Curtis, and S. Hammill. "Non-evidence-based ICD Implantations in the United States." *Journal of the American Medical Association* 305, no. 1 (2011): 43–49. doi:10.1001/jama.2010.1915.

Rate of unnecessary cesarean sections:

Gibbons, L., J. M. Belizán, J. A., Lauer, A. P. Betrán, M. Merialdi, and F. Althabe. "The Global Numbers and Costs of Additionally Needed and Unnecessary Caesarean Sections Performed Per Year: Overuse as a Barrier to Universal Coverage." *World Health Report (2010) Background Paper*, no. 30 (2010). https://www.who.int/healthsystems/topics/financing/healthreport/30C-sectioncosts.pdf.

Number of c-sections in the US:

Martin, J. A., B. E. Hamilton, M. J. K. Osterman, A. K. Driscoll, and P. Drake. "Births: Final data for 2016." *National Vital Statistics Reports* 67, no. 1 (2018): 1–55.

Waste in US healthcare system:

Shrank, W. H., T. L. Rogstad, and N. Parekh. "Waste in US Healthcare System: Estimated Costs and Potential for Savings." *Journal of the American Medical Association* (October 7, 2019), early release. doi: 10.1001/jama.2019.13978.

Unnecessary tests and procedures:

Gawande, A. "Overkill." *The New Yorker*, May 11, 2015. https://www.newyorker.com/magazine/2015/05/11/overkill-atul-gawande.

CHAPTER 22

Physician suicide:

Anderson, P. "Physicians Experience Highest Suicide Rate of Any Profession." *Medscape* (May 7, 2018). https://www.medscape.com/viewarticle/896257#vp_1.

Farmer, B. "When Doctors Struggle with Suicide, Their Profession Often Fails Them." *Morning Edition*, National Public Radio, July 31, 2018. https://www.npr.org/sections/health-shots/2018/07/31/634217947/to-prevent-doctor-suicides-medical-industry-rethinks-how-doctors-work.

García Márquez story and Willa Cather quote:

Cather, Willa. *My Mortal Enemy.* New York: Vintage Books, 1954.

García Márquez, G. *Chronicle of a Death Foretold.* Translated by Gregory Rabassa. New York: Vintage International Edition, 2003.

EPILOGUE

Empathy improves patients' lives and outcomes:

Dacely, J., and A. Fotopolou. "Why Empathy has a Beneficial Impact on Others in Medicine; Unifying Theories." *Frontiers in Behavioral Neuroscience* 8 (2014): 457.

Derksen, F., J. Bensing, and A. Lagroz-Janssen. "Effectiveness of Empathy in General Practice: A Systematic Review." *British Journal of General Practice* 63, no. 606 (2013): e76–e84.

Street, R. L., Jr., G. Makoul, N. K. Arora, and R. M. Epstein. "How Does Communication Heal? Pathways Linking Clinician–patient Communication to Health Outcomes." *Patient Education and Counseling* 74, no. 3 (2009): 295–301.

Nurturing empathy, and doctor as a patient:

Rahman, F. "Nurturing Empathy: An Oncologist Looks at Medicine and Himself." *The Oncologist* 19 (2014): 1287–88.

A medical student with cancer and his difficulty with the role as a patient—roles reversed:

Hardison, S. A. "A New Reality." *Annals of Internal Medicine* 156, no. 4 (2012): 319–20.

Value of teaching medical humanities to students and doctors:

Carver, R. "What the Doctor Said." In *All of US: The Collected Poems*, edited by William Stull. New York: Vintage, 2015. Ebook edition.

Chekhov, A. "Ward No. 6." In *The Essential Tales of Chekhov*, edited by Richard Ford. New York: Ecco Press, 1998.

Arthur Horwich quote:

Devi, S. "Lasker Foundation Honors Malaria Researcher." *The Lancet* 378 (2011): 1129.

Susan Sontag quote:

Sontag, S. *Illness as Metaphor and AIDS and its Metaphors*. New York: First Picador USA edition, 2001, 3.

Racial disparities in cancer pain control and cancer care:

Enzinger, A. C., K. Ghosh, N. L. Keating, et al. "Racial and Ethnic Disparities in Opioid Access and Urine Drug Screening Among Older Patients with Poor-prognosis Cancer Near the End of Life." *Journal of Clinical Oncology* 41, no. 14 (January 10, 2023). dol:10.1200/ JCO.22.0413.

Lillard, J. W., Jr, K. A. Moses, B. A. Mahal, et al. "Racial Disparities in Black Men with Prostate Cancer: A Literature Review." *Cancer* 128 (2022): 3787–95.

Liou, K. T. "Addressing Racial Disparities in Cancer Pain Management: A Potential Role for Music Therapy." *The ASCO Post*, June 10, 2023. https://ascopost.com/news/april-2023/addressing-racial-dispari-ties-in-cancer-pain-management-a-potential-role-for-music-therapy/.

Patients prefer personal contact with doctors, survey:

McBride, Aloha. "The EY Global Consumer Health Survey 2023 Finds Consumers Value Access Most, but Also Want Cost-Effective Care and Relief from Pain and Anxiety." www.ey.com/en_us/health/ ey-consumer-health-survey-2023.

Palliative care:

Helwick, C. "How Effectively Are You Helping Patients with Cancer at the End of Life?" *The ASCO Post*, April 25, 2023. https://ascopost.com/ issues/april-25-2023/ how-effectively-are-you-helping-patients-with-cancer-at-the-end-of-life/.

Wealthy nonprofit hospitals:

Kliff, S., and J. Silver-Greenberg. "This Non-profit Health System Cuts Off Patients with Medical Debt." *New York Times*, June 1, 2023.

CPR in the debilitated elderly:

Rahman, F. "Why Pound Life into the Dying?" *New York Times,* February 20, 1989.

Struggling to care for the oldest old:

Winakur, J. *Memory Lessons: A Doctor's Story.* New York: Hyperion, 2009.

NOTE: *The ASCO Post* is a free online and print magazine that publishes the latest news on research, diagnosis, and treatment of cancer and is a reliable source of information. Although the magazine is aimed at oncologists, it also frequently publishes stories on economic, social, and global aspects of cancer care and cancer patients' own personal experiences. It's a publication of the American Society of Clinical Oncology (ASCO), a worldwide professional organization of cancer doctors of all oncology subspecialties, including medical, surgical, radiation, and research oncology. In addition, Cancer.Net from ASCO is a good source of free information for cancer patients and their families and caregivers. (Disclosure: I am a member of ASCO, and I was once on its Clinical Practice Committee and Subcommittee on Pain Control.)

INDEX

ABOUT THE AUTHOR

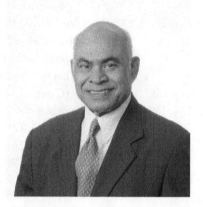

F azlur Rahman was born and brought up in what is now Bangladesh. After his medical education in Dhaka, New York, and Houston, he practiced cancer medicine for thirty-five years in San Angelo, Texas. He is an adjunct professor of biology (medical humanities and ethics) at Angelo State University, a senior trustee of Austin College in Sherman, Texas, and an advisory council member of the Charles E. Cheever Jr. Center for Medical Humanities and Ethics at the University of Texas Health Science Center in San Antonio.

His writings on medical, ethical, social, and scientific issues have appeared in many national and international publications, including the *New York Times, Wall Street Journal, Guardian Weekly, International Herald Tribune, Haaretz, Indian Express, Christian Science Monitor, Newsweek, Harvard Review, Short Story International, Dallas Morning News, Houston Chronicle, Oncologist,* and *Lancet.* His cultural and medical memoir, *The Temple Road: A Doctor's Journey,* published in India in 2016, tells about his upbringing and training years, his move to a new country, and his life and practice in West Texas. He and his wife, Jahanara (Ara), have lived there for most of their lives and have raised four children. They love walking in nature and going on wildflower adventures.